HEALTH, HARM or RIP-OFF?

What's REALLY in Your Vitamins & Supplements

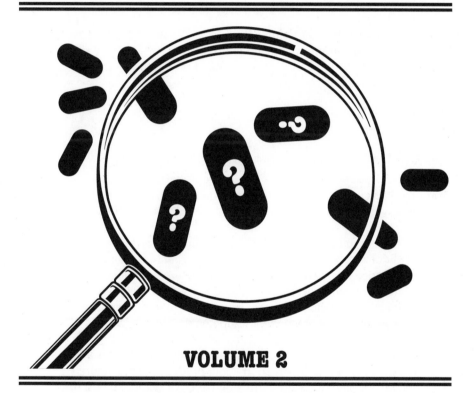

VOLUME 2

ConsumerLab.com's Inside Guide to More Than 800 Products

Edited by Tod Cooperman, M.D.

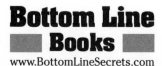

Bottom Line Books

www.BottomLineSecrets.com

HEALTH, HARM or RIP-OFF? Volume 2
What's Really in Your Vitamins and Supplements
ConsumerLab.com's Inside Guide to More Than 800 Products
Edited by Tod Cooperman, M.D.

Deluxe two-volume edition of *ConsumerLab.com's Guide to Buying Vitamins and Supplements: What's Really in the Bottle?* by the staff of ConsumerLab.com; edited by Tod Cooperman, M.D., published by arrangement with ConsumerLab.com, LLC, White Plains, NY 10605

Information in this guide is provided for informational purposes only. It is not an endorsement of any product nor is it meant to substitute for the advice provided by physicians or other health care professionals. The information contained herein should not be used for diagnosing or treating a health problem or disease. Consumers should inform their health care providers of the dietary supplements they take.

The reviews published in this guide are based on label evaluations and analytic testing. Names and information about products, manufacturers and distributors, or other factual information were correct to the best of our knowledge when incorporated into this guide; any subsequent changes may not be reflected.

Bottom Line Books® is a registered trademark of Boardroom® Inc., 281 Tresser Blvd., Stamford, CT 06901   www.BottomLineSecrets.com

ISBN   0-88723-450-X

10   9   8   7   6   5   4   3   2   1

Printed in the United States of America

Contents

Contents

Part 3
Product Reviews: Herbal Supplements

Contents

Part 8
Product Screening

Appendices

Part 4

Product Reviews:
Vitamins & Minerals

B Vitamins: Thiamin, Niacin, B-6, B-12, Riboflavin, and Folic Acid

The eight B vitamins are individually known as thiamin hydrochloride (B-1), riboflavin (B-2), niacin (B-3), pantothenic acid (B-5), pyridoxine hydrochloride (B-6), cyanocobalamin (B-12), folic acid (folate) and biotin. Like most vitamins, B vitamins are essential; your body cannot make them, and you must get them from your diet or supplements.

Each B vitamin is associated with a variety of functions. Several (B-6, B-12, and folic acid) have shown promise for reducing the risk of heart disease, leading to the current popularity of B complex supplements. Folic acid is also important in reducing birth defects of the spinal cord and is, therefore, a critical ingredient in prenatal vitamins. Niacin, when taken in very high doses, can improve cholesterol levels. (See ConsumerTips™ for Buying and Using, page 318, for more information on uses, doses, safe levels, and food sources for each of the B vitamins.)

Quality Concerns and Product Testing

Earlier research by ConsumerLab.com had found problems with the B vitamin content of several supplements. Neither the U.S. government nor any agency is responsible for routinely testing B vitamin products or other dietary supplements for their contents or quality.

ConsumerLab.com, as part of its mission to independently evaluate products that affect health, wellness, and nutrition, purchased dietary supplements sold in the U.S. and Canada claiming to contain single B vitamins or B vitamin complexes. These products were tested to see if they contained their claimed amounts of the eight B vitamins. Products sold as tablets or caplets were also tested for their ability to break apart properly for absorption. In addition, products were evaluated to determine if their suggested daily dose exceeded Tolerable Upper Intake Levels (UL) for B vitamins as established by the Institute of Medicine of the National Academies. (See the appropriate section in "ConsumerLab.com's Testing Methods and Standards," page 653, in the appendix for more details about the testing.)

Test Findings

ConsumerLab.com selected, purchased, and tested 16 B vitamin supplements. Four of these were B vitamin complexes and the others contained single B vitamins: two with B-6, three with B-12, three with niacin (B-3), two with folic acid, one with thiamin (B-1), and one with biotin.

Of these products, one failed testing for the following reasons: Mega Food® Balanced B Complex was short on its folic acid—only 330 mcg per pill rather than the claimed 400 micrograms (mcg). Folic acid is taken to help prevent birth defects (400 mcg is recommended daily from a supplement during pregnancy) and it may work along with B-6 to reduce the risk of heart disease and strokes in adults.

All of the products that were in tablet or caplet form were able to disintegrate (break apart) properly, as needed for absorption.

ConsumerLab.com found that the recommended doses of all the niacin-only products and many of the B complex products exceeded established Tolerable Upper Intake Levels (UL) for adults for niacin, above which there is increased risk of side effects with regular use. The adult UL for niacin is 35 milligrams (mg) per day. Doses much higher than the UL are used medically to improve cholesterol levels. However, high doses of niacin can cause dangerous liver inflammation. For this reason, regular lab tests and the supervision of a healthcare professional are strongly advised before taking niacin at doses above the UL. (See ConsumerTips™ for Buying and Using below for more information about potential side effects with various forms of niacin.)

The 16 products that were selected for testing and a summary of the results are listed alphabetically in Test Results for B-Vitamin Supplements. Also included in the list are 25 other products (indicated with an asterisk) that have met the same criteria through CL's Voluntary Certification Program (see Selection and Testing, page 25, volume 1). Those products that exceeded recommendations on safe upper levels (ULs) for certain ingredients are indicated with an explanatory footnote.

ConsumerTips™ for Buying and Using

ConsumerLab.com has prepared numerous important tips about dosing, selecting, and buy B vitamin supplements. This information, along with our list of approved brands, provides a valuable guide for choosing appropriate products. Information in "The Bs" will help you determine the amounts appropriate for your gender and life stage.

DRI's Reviewed

Be sure that you are getting enough B vitamins to meet basic nutrient requirements and avoid deficiencies. Check the recommended intakes listed for each. These values, known as Dietary Reference Intakes (DRI), are established by the Institute of Medicine of the National Academies. One type of DRI is a Recommended Dietary Allowance (RDA), which is the average daily dietary intake level that is sufficient to meet the nutrient requirement of nearly all healthy individuals in a particular life stage and gender. Another type of DRI is an Adequate Intake (AI), which is similar to an RDA but is more of an approximation used when not enough sufficient information is available to develop an RDA. As required by the FDA, dietary supplement labels or packages must show the percent of the Daily Value for certain vitamins and minerals that they contain. However, the percentages given may not reflect the latest Recommended Dietary Allowances (RDA) or Adequate Intakes (AI).

If you are buying B vitamins to treat a specific medical condition, such as high cholesterol, or to try to reduce the risk of heart disease, you will generally need more than the recommended intakes. Look at each vitamin for suggested doses for treating specific conditions.

In either case, be aware that you can get too much of some vitamins. A Tolerable Upper Intake Level (UL) is the highest level of daily intake of a nutrient that is likely to pose no risk of adverse health effects for most people. As intakes increase above the UL, the risk of adverse effects may increase. Like the RDA and AI, the UL vary according to age and gender. Individuals are advised not to regularly exceed the UL, unless the amount is medically recommended and the intake is supervised. Be aware that products are not required to provide information indicating whether their ingredients may exceed UL for the individuals for whom they are intended. As discovered by ConsumerLab.com, many do exceed these UL.

Most products will list the amount of each ingredient. The information provided with the Bs can help you to determine whether such amounts are appropriate. Keep in mind that 1,000 mcg (micrograms) is the same as 1 mg (milligram), and 1,000 mg equals 1 gram.

The Bs

Thiamin Hydrochloride (B-1): Thiamin assists the nervous system. It is found in large enough amounts in yeast, peas, beans, and grains that if these foods are regularly included in your diet, supplementation is normally not necessary. Thiamin deficiency, however, can occur in people taking strong diuretics (loop diuretics) for congestive heart failure, and this deficiency itself can adversely affect heart function. Thiamin deficiency is also common in people who abuse alcohol.

Recommended intake: The RDA is 0.5 mg for children 1 to 3, 0.6 mg for those 4 to 8, and 0.9 mg for those 9 to 13. For males ages 14 and older, the RDA is 1.2 mg. For females ages 14 to 18, the RDA is 1.0 mg, and it increases to 1.1 mg for those 19 and older. However, the RDA for pregnant or lactating women is 1.4 mg. For use to counter the effects of diuretics, a dose of 100 mg twice daily has been used.

Upper limit: No UL has been established for thiamine. This appears to be a nontoxic supplement.

Riboflavin (B-2): Riboflavin maintains vision and skin. Although found in many vegetables and nuts, some supplementation may be needed in children and the elderly.

Recommended intake: The RDA is 0.5 mg for children 1 to 3, 0.6 mg for those 4 to 8, and 0.9 mg for those 9 to 13. For males ages 14 and older, the RDA is 1.3 mg. For females ages 14 to 18, the RDA is 1.0 mg, and it increases to 1.1 mg for those 19 and older. However, the RDA for pregnant women is 1.4 mg, and for lactating women, it is 1.6 mg. Much higher amounts (400 mg a day) have been suggested in the prevention of migraines.

Upper limit: No UL has been established for riboflavin.

Niacin (B-3): Also known as nicotinic acid, niacin helps release energy from carbohydrates and is available in the diet from enriched white flour as well as peanuts, fish, and meat. When taken in very high doses, it can help improve cholesterol levels and, thereby, reduce death rates from cardiovascular disease. A modified form of niacin called inositol hexanicotinate (or hexaniacinate) is said to cause less flushing than regular niacin, and it may reduce cholesterol levels. In addition to reducing cholesterol levels, niacin has been studied particularly as a treatment for intermittent claudication (a kind of leg cramping caused by hardening of the arteries) as well as for Raynaud's disease (another condition that involves arterial blood flow). Niacinamide (or nicotinamide) is another form of niacin; it does not lower cholesterol, but it has been proposed for helping to prevent diabetes in children who are at risk for developing it. (Unfortunately, the results of recent studies have not been promising.)

Recommended intake: The RDA is 6 mg for children 1 to 3, 8 mg for those 4 to 8, and 12 mg for those 9 to 13. For males ages 14 and older, the RDA is 16 mg. For females ages 14 and older, the RDA is 14 mg. However, the RDA for pregnant women is 18 mg, and for lactating women, it is 17 mg. Niacin has shown effects for improving cholesterol profiles, but only when taken in doses that are far higher than the RDA and UL—ranging from 1,000 mg to 4,000 mg (1 to 4 grams) per day. Liver injury is a real possibility when niacin is used in this way. Be aware that the amount of niacin in inositol hexanicotinate is about 85%; therefore, if the front of the bottle says 600 mg inositol hexanicotinate, the product should be expected to have about 500 mg of niacin.

Upper limit: Daily doses over 50 mg a day have been associated with flushing of the skin, including reddening, burning, tingling, itching, and pain. Starting with a lower dose and then gradually increasing it may reduce this side effect, as may taking the supplement with food. Slow-release niacin and products made from nicotinamide (or niacinamide) and inositol hexanicotinate are also less likely to cause the flushing reaction. However, at doses over 1,500 mg (1.5 grams) of niacin or 3,000 mg (3 grams) of nicotinamide a day liver toxicity can occur and may be more common among people taking slow-release niacin (though it is also possible that the flushing side effect simply makes many people unable to use high dosages of ordinary niacin). The UL for niacin applies only to that consumed from supplements and fortified foods (naturally occurring food sources are not included) and is 10 mg for children 1 to 3, 15 mg for those 4 to 8, 20 mg for those 9 to 13, 30 mg for those 14 to 18, and 35 mg for individuals 19 years and older. *Caution:* Niacinamide may increase blood levels of anticonvulsant drugs.

Pantothenic Acid (B-5): Pantothenic acid is involved in the production of energy as well as the synthesis of hormones and neurotransmitters. Deficiency is rare (although seen in alcoholics), and it is found in many foods, with particularly high levels in liver, yeast, and salmon.

Recommended intake: The AI is 2 mg for children 1 to 3, 3 mg for children 4 to 8, and 4 mg for children 9 to 13. For individuals ages 14 and older, the AI is 5 mg. However, the AI for pregnant women is 6 mg, and for women who breastfeed, it is 7 mg. Much higher doses

(900 mg a day) of the related substance pantothenate have been used in improving cholesterol profiles (especially reducing triglyceride levels).

Upper limit: No UL has been established for pantothenic acid.

Pyridoxine Hydrochloride (B-6): Pyridoxine hydrochloride is important in many aspects of metabolism and in maintaining the immune and nervous systems. Pyridoxine in amounts that meet the RDAs is easily available from your diet; however, mild deficiency is common, particularly in the elderly and children.

Recommended intake: The RDA is 0.5 mg for children 1 to 3, 0.6 mg for those 4 to 8, and 1.0 mg for those 9 to 13. For males ages 14 to 50, the RDA is 1.3 mg, and for those 51 and older, it is 1.7 mg. For females ages 14 to 18, it is 1.2 mg; for those 19 to 50, it is 1.3 mg; and for those 51 and older, it is 1.5 mg. However, the RDA for pregnant women is 1.9 mg, and for lactating women, it is 2.0 mg. Amounts higher than the RDA but lower than the UL have been recommended to help reduce the risk of heart disease (5 to 30 mg/day) and to help reduce the nausea of morning sickness (30 mg/day); some evidence supports these uses. Other proposed uses of pyridoxine, such as treating asthma, autism, carpal tunnel syndrome, diabetic neuropathy, tardive dyskinesia, and PMS, may involve doses higher than the UL; however, none of these uses has good scientific support.

Upper limit: Too much pyridoxine can cause nerve damage and skin lesions. These effects are generally seen at doses over 1,000 mg a day, though rare cases have been seen at 200 mg daily. The UL for pyridoxine is 30 mg for children ages 1 to 3, 40 mg for those 4 to 8, 60 mg for those 9 to 13, 80 mg for those 14 to 18, and 100 mg for individuals ages 19 and older.

Folic Acid (B-9, folate): Also known as folate and folacin, folic acid reduces the risk of spina bifida in offspring (a leading cause of childhood paralysis) when consumed by pregnant women. Folic acid may also reduce the chance of other birth defects as well as childhood leukemia in offspring, and it may work along with B-6 to reduce the risk of heart disease and strokes in adults. Good sources of folic acid include dark green leafy vegetables such as spinach, kale, and collards, and oranges. Most people can get sufficient folic acid from their diet, but supplements are generally recommended for women who are pregnant or may soon become pregnant.

Recommended intake: It is important to know, however, that the RDA are based on intake from regular food sources. Folic acid from supplements and fortified foods is actually absorbed twice as well as that from regular food sources. Consequently, if you are relying on supplements or fortified foods to reach the RDA, you need only one-half the amount listed in the following RDA: 150 mcg for children ages 1 to 3, 200 mcg for children 4 to 8, and 300 mcg for children 9 to 13. For individuals ages 14 and older, the RDA is 400 mcg. However, the RDA for pregnant women is 600 mcg, and for lactating women, it is 500 mcg. In view of its importance to developing fetuses during the first few weeks after conception, all women capable of becoming pregnant should consume 400 mcg from supplements or fortified foods, in addition to intake of folic acid from a varied diet.

Upper limit: Prolonged intake of excessive folic acid can cause kidney damage and can complicate the diagnosis of vitamin B-12 deficiency. The UL for folic acid applies only to that consumed from supplements and fortified foods and is 300 mcg for children ages 1 to 3, 400 mcg for those 4 to 8, 600 mcg for those 9 to 13, and 800 mcg for those 14 to 18. For individuals ages 19 and older, the UL is 1,000 mcg.

Cyanocobalamin (B-12): Cyanocobalamin deficiency

can cause anemia, irreversible nerve damage, and low sperm count. B-12 has been used along with vitamin B-6 in reducing the risk of heart disease. Vitamin B-12 is found in abundant quantity in meats and is also plentiful in poultry and fish but not found in plant foods. A healthful diet should meet the vitamin B-12 RDA, but supplementation is often needed for strict vegetarians, alcohol and drug abusers, people recovering from surgery or burns, or those with bowel or pancreatic cancer. Deficiency may also occur in people with low stomach acidity, such as older individuals or those taking medications that reduce stomach acid, because stomach acid is necessary to allow absorption of vitamin B-12 from foods. The purified vitamin B-12 found in supplements does not require stomach acid for absorption. Consequently, it is advisable for people over 50 years of age as well as those taking medications such as Prilosec or Zantac to meet their RDA by consuming foods fortified with purified vitamin B-12 or by taking a dietary supplement.

Recommended intake: The RDA is 0.9 mcg for children ages 1 to 3, 1.2 mcg for those 4 to 8, and 1.8 mcg for those 9 to 13. For individuals ages 14 and older, the RDA is 2.4 mcg. However, the RDA for pregnant women is 2.6 mcg and for lactating women, it is 2.8 mcg. Higher doses of vitamin B-12 (about 400 mcg a day) have been proposed for helping to prevent heart disease. Vitamin B-12 in far higher dosages has also been proposed for the treatment of other conditions including asthma, fatigue, and male infertility, but there is no reliable evidence that it is effective.

Upper Limit: No UL has been established for vitamin B-12. This appears to be a very safe ingredient.

Biotin: Biotin is needed for the metabolism of nutrients. Deficiency is rare under normal circumstances because biotin can be produced in the gut by bacteria and is also found in organ meats, oatmeal, egg yolk, mushrooms, bananas, peanuts, and brewer's yeast. However, deficiency might occur with long-term use of antibiotics or antiseizure medications. Note: Biotin might impair the absorption of some antiseizure medications, and for this reason, people taking such medications should use biotin supplements only under the supervision of a healthcare professional.

Recommended intake: The AI for biotin is 8 mcg for children ages 1 to 3, 12 mcg for those 4 to 8, and 20 mcg for those 9 to 13. For individuals ages 14 to 18, the AI is 25 mcg, and for those 19 and older, it is 30 mcg. However, the AI increases to 35 mcg for women who are breast-feeding.

Upper Limit: No UL has been established for biotin.

Concerns and Cautions

Try to avoid taking too much of any B vitamin. Check the UL, and if you need to take a product with vitamins exceeding the UL, do so under a physician's supervision and with awareness of potential side effects.

Be aware that certain B vitamins can interact with other drugs and supplements as noted.

Test Results for B-Vitamin Supplements

Product (label info: suggested serving)‡ Manufacturer (Mf) or distributor (Dist)	Test Results		
	Approved or not approved	Contained labeled amounts of B vitamins (See B Vitamins: Label Amounts, page 334)	Broke apart properly
B-Complex			
CVS® Pharmacy Vitamin Super B Complex & C (1 caplet/day)* Dist: CVS Pharmacy, Inc	approved	✔	✔
Enzymatic Therapy Natural Medicines® Fatigued to Fantastic Daily Energy B Complex (1 capsule/day)* Mf: Enzymatic Therapy, Inc.	approved	✔	N/A
Healthy Moments™ Margarita Lime Flavor Vitamin Strips, B-Complex for Energy (1 strip/day) Dist: Momentus Solutions, LLC	approved	✔	N/A
Mega Food® Balanced B Complex Daily Foods® Vitamin Formula, 100% Whole Food, Vegetarian Formula (1 tablet/day) Mf: Mega Food	**not** approved	Contained only 82% of labeled amount of folic acid	✔

continued

Product (label info.)	Test Results		
	Approval	Contained labeled	Broke apart
Nature Made® Super B-Complex Supplement with Vitamin C, with Folic Acid, USP (1 tablet/day)* Dist: Nature Made Nutritional Products	approved	✔	✔
Nature's Bounty® Time Released B Complex Vitamins plus Vitamin C (1 tablet/day)* Mf: Nature's Bounty, Inc.	approved	✔	N/A
🏃 Pharmanex® LifePak® Dietary Supplement, New! Anti-Aging Formula (1 packet/day)* Dist: Pharmanex, LLC	approved; also approved for alpha-lipoic acid, multi-vitamins, vitamin C and vitamin E	✔	N/A
Pioneer® Vegetarian B-Complex Stress Formula, with Herbs & Coenzymes (2 tablets/day) Dist: Pioneer Nutritional Formulas, Inc.	approved	✔	✔
Puritan's Pride® B-100® Ultra B-Complex (1 tablet/day)* Mf: Puritan's Pride, Inc.	approved	✔	✔

Product (label info.)	Test Results		
	Approval	Contained labeled	Broke apart
Puritan's Pride® B-50® B-Complex Vitamin (1 tablet/day)* Mf: Puritan's Pride, Inc.	approved	✔	✔
Sundown® Benefits B Super Maxi Complex (1 caplet/day)* Dist: Rexall Sundown, Inc.	approved	✔	✔
TwinLab® B-50 Caps Vitamin B-Complex Dietary Supplement (1 capsule/day) Dist: Twin Laboratories Inc.	approved***	✔	N/A
Vitamin World® B-Complex Sublingual Liquid (1 mL/day)* Mf: Vitamin World, Inc.	approved	✔	N/A
Vitamin World® Naturally Inspired™ B-100® Ultra B-Complex (1 tablet/ day)* Mf: Vitamin World, Inc	approved	✔	✔

continued

Product (label info.)	Test Results		
	Approval	Contained labeled	Broke apart
B-1 (Thiamin)			
Bluebonnet Vitamin B-1 100 mg (1 vegetarian capsule/day) Mf: Bluebonnet Nutrition Corporation	approved**	✔	N/A
B-3 (Niacin)			
Nature's Bounty Flush Free Niacin (1 capsule/day)* Mf: Nature's Bounty, Inc	approved	✔	N/A
Puritan's Pride® Flush Free Niacin Inositol Hexanicotinate 500 mg (1 capsule/day)* Mf: Puritan's Pride, Inc	approved	✔	N/A
Rite Aid Niacin 100 mg (1 tablet/day) Dist: Rite Aid Corporation	approved	✔	✔
Slo Niacin®, polygel® controlled-release niacin (1 tablet/day) Dist: Upsher-Smith Laboratories, Inc.	approved	✔	N/A

Product (label info.)	Test Results		
	Approval	Contained labeled	Broke apart
Thorne Research Niacinamide (1 vegetarian capsule/ day) Mf: Thorne Research, Inc.	approved	✔	N/A
Vitamin World® Naturally Inspired™ Flush Free Niacin, Inositol Hexanicotinate 500 mg (1 capsule/ day)* Mf: Vitamin World, Inc.	approved	✔	N/A
B-6 (Pyridoxine)			
Akyma Pharmaceuticals Vitamin B-6 (Pyridoxine HCl) 50 mg (1 tablet/day) Dist: Akyma Pharmaceuticals LLC	approved	✔	✔
Mason natural® Vitamin B Supplement B-6 100 mg (1 tablet/ day) Dist: Mason Vitamins, Inc.	approved	✔	✔
Puritan's Pride® Vitamin B-6 100 mg (1 tablet/day)* Mf: Puritan's Pride, Inc.	approved	✔	✔

continued

Product (label info.)	Test Results		
	Approval	Contained labeled	Broke apart
B-12			
Country Life® Hypoallergenic Vitamin B-12 500 mcg (1 tablet/day) Mf: Country Life	approved	✔	✔
Equaline™ High Potency 1000 mcg Vitamin B-12, Natural, Time Release (1 tablet/day) Dist: Albertsons, Inc.	approved	✔	N/A
Puritan's Pride® Sublingual B-12 Microlozenges 500 mcg (1 microlozenge/day)* Mf: Puritan's Pride, Inc.	approved	✔	N/A
Puritan's Pride® Time Release Vitamin B-12 1000 mcg ENER-B® (1 tablet/day)* Mf: Puritan's Pride, Inc.	approved	✔	N/A
Rexall® Sublingual High Potency B-12 2500 mcg (1 microlozenge/day)* Mf: Rexall, Inc.	approved	✔	N/A

Product (label info.)	Test Results		
	Approval	Contained labeled	Broke apart
SISU Vitamin B-12 1000 mcg (1 capsule/day) Mf: SISU Inc.	approved	✔	N/A
Sundown® Benefits B12 High Potency 1000 mcg (1 tablet/ day)* Mf: Sundown Inc.	approved	✔	✔
Vitamin World® Naturally Inspired™ Sublingual B-12 Microlozenges 500 mcg (1 microlozenge/day)* Mf: Vitamin World, Inc.	approved	✔	N/A
Vitamin World® Naturally Inspired™ Time Release Vitamin B-12 1000 mcg (1 tablet/day)* Dist: Vitamin World, Inc.	approved	✔	N/A
Vitamin World® Naturally Inspired™ Sublingual Vitamin B-12 5000 mcg (1 lozenge/day)* Mf: Vitamin World, Inc	approved	✔	N/A

continued

331

Product (label info.)	Test Results		
	Approval	Contained labeled	Broke apart
Biotin			
Nature's Bounty® High Potency Biotin 1000 mcg (1 tablet/ day)* Mf: Nature's Bounty, Inc.	approved	✔	✔
Nature's Life® Biotin 2,500 mcg (1 capsule/ day) Dist: Nature's Life	approved	✔	N/A
Puritan's Pride® Super Biotin 5000 mcg (1 capsule/day)* Mf: Puritan's Pride, Inc.	approved	✔	N/A
Rexall® Extreme Biotin 1500 mcg (1 tablet/ day)* Mf: Rexall, Inc.	approved	✔	✔
Vitamin World® Naturally Inspired™ Super Biotin 5000 mcg (1 capsule/day)* Mf: Vitamin World, Inc.	approved	✔	N/A
Folic Acid			
Natural Factors® Folic Acid 1 mg, Plus 20 mg C (1 tablet/day) Dist: Natural Factors	approved	✔	✔

Product (label info.)	Test Results		
	Approval	Contained labeled	Broke apart
Puritan's Pride® Folic Acid 800 mcg (1 tablet/day)* Mf: Puritan's Pride, Inc.	approved	✔	✔
🍁Swiss™ Natural Sources Folic Acid 1 mg Plus, USP (1 tablet/day) Dist: Swiss Herbal Remedies Ltd.	approved	✔	✔

*Tested through CL's Voluntary Certification Program before, at the time of, or after the initial review.

**The status of this product was updated to "Approved" on 4/30/05. Originally reported as "Not Approved." Re-analysis found the amount of thiamin to be correctly labeled.

***The status of this product was updated to "Approved" on 6/13/05. Originally reported as "Not Approved." Re-analysis found the amount of riboflavin (as riboflavin-5-phosphate [sodium]), to be correctly labeled.

N/A—Not applicable: Disintegration test applies only to tablets and caplets. Not applicable to chewable products, powders, capsules, liquid, and time-release forms.

✔ Check indicates the results met the criteria listed in the column heading.

‡ See also "More Brand Information," page 675.

🏃 Product passed optional Athletic Banned Screening Program

🍁 Purchased from a retailer in Canada.

B Vitamins: Label Amounts

Product (label info: Mf suggested serving)‡ Manufacturer (Mf) or Distributor (Dist)	Labeled amount of B vitamins		
	B-1[a] (mg)	B-2[b] (mg)	B-3[c] (mg)
B-Complex			
CVS® Pharmacy Vitamin Super B Complex & C (1 caplet/day)* Dist: CVS Pharmacy, Inc	100	20	25
Enzymatic Therapy Natural Medicines® Fatigued to Fantastic Daily Energy B Complex (1 capsule/day)* Mf: Enzymatic Therapy, Inc.	75	75	50[1]
Healthy Moments™ Margarita Lime Flavor Vitamin Strips, B-Complex for Energy (1 strip/day) Dist: Healthy Moments	1.2	1.2	N/A
Mega Food® Balanced B Complex Daily Foods® Vitamin Formula, 100% Whole Food, Vegetarian Formula (1 tablet/day) Mf: Mega Food	11	9	30

B-5[d] (mg)	B-6[e] (mg)	B-12[f] (mcg)	Biotin (mg)	Folic acid (mcg)
5.5	2	15	5	400
50	85	500	N/A	800
5	1.3	2.4	N/A	N/A
23	11	125	300	400

continued

Product (label info.)	Labeled amount of B vitamins		
	B-1[a] (mg)	B-2[b] (mg)	B-3[c] (mg)
Nature Made® Super B-Complex Supplement with Vitamin C, with Folic Acid, USP (1 tablet/ day)* Dist: Nature Made Nutritional Products	100	20	25
Nature's Bounty® Time Released B Complex Vitamins plus Vitamin C (1 tablet/day)* Mf: Nature's Bounty, Inc.	18	10	50[1]
🏃 Pharmanex® LifePak® Dietary Supplement, New! Anti-Aging Formula (1 packet/day)* Dist: Pharmanex, LLC	3.75	4.25	20[1]
Pioneer® Vegetarian B-Complex Stress Formula, with Herbs & Coenzymes (2 tablets/day) Dist: Pioneer Nutritional Formulas, Inc.	25	25	37.5[1]
Puritan's Pride® B-100® Ultra B-Complex (1 tablet/ day)* Mf: Puritan's Pride, Inc.	100	100	100[1]

B-5[d] (mg)	B-6[e] (mg)	B-12[f] (mcg)	Biotin (mg)	Folic acid (mcg)
5.5	2	15	30	400
10	5	10	50	400
15	5	15	N/A	300
125	25	125	150	500
100	100	100	100	400

continued

Product (label info.)	Labeled amount of B vitamins		
	B-1[a] (mg)	B-2[b] (mg)	B-3[c] (mg)
Puritan's Pride® B-50® B-Complex Vitamin (1 tablet/ day)* Mf: Puritan's Pride, Inc.	50	50	50[1]
Sundown® Benefits B Super Maxi Complex (1 caplet/day)* Dist: Rexall Sundown, Inc.	15	17	200[1]
TwinLab® B-50 Caps Vitamin B-Complex Dietary Supplement (1 capsule/day) Dist: Twin Laboratories Inc.	50	50	50[1]
Vitamin World® B-Complex Sublingual Liquid (1 mL/day)* Mf: Vitamin World, Inc.	N/A	1.7	20
Vitamin World® Naturally Inspired™ B-100® Ultra B-Complex (1 tablet/ day)* Mf: Vitamin World, Inc	100	100	100[1]

B-5[d] (mg)	B-6[e] (mg)	B-12[f] (mcg)	Biotin (mg)	Folic acid (mcg)
50	50	50	50	400
100	20	60	N/A	400
50	50	50	50	400
30	2	1200	N/A	N/A
100	100	100	100	400

continued

Product (label info.)	Labeled amount of B vitamins		
	B-1[a] (mg)	B-2[b] (mg)	B-3[c] (mg)
B-1 (Thiamin)			
Bluebonnet Vitamin B-1 100 mg (1 vegetarian capsule/day) Mf: Bluebonnet Nutrition Corporation	100	N/A	N/A
B-3 (Niacin)			
Nature's Bounty Flush Free Niacin (1 capsule/day)* Mf: Nature's Bounty, Inc	N/A	N/A	400[1]
Puritan's Pride® Flush Free Niacin Inositol Hexanicotinate 500 mg (1 capsule/day)* Mf: Puritan's Pride, Inc.	N/A	N/A	400[1]
Rite Aid Niacin 100 mg (1 tablet/ day) Dist: Rite Aid Corporation	N/A	N/A	100[1]
Slo Niacin®, polygel® controlled-release niacin (1 tablet/day) Dist: Upsher-Smith Laboratories, Inc.	N/A	N/A	250[1]

B-5[d] (mg)	B-6[e] (mg)	B-12[f] (mcg)	Biotin (mg)	Folic acid (mcg)
N/A	N/A	N/A	N/A	N/A
N/A	N/A	N/A	N/A	N/A
N/A	N/A	N/A	N/A	N/A
N/A	N/A	N/A	N/A	N/A
N/A	N/A	N/A	N/A	N/A

continued

Product (label info.)	Labeled amount of B vitamins		
	B-1[a] (mg)	B-2[b] (mg)	B-3[c] (mg)
Thorne Research Niacinamide (1 vegetarian capsule/day) Mf: Thorne Research, Inc.	N/A	N/A	500[1]
Vitamin World® Naturally Inspired™ Flush Free Niacin, Inositol Hexanicotinate 500 mg (1 capsule/ day)* Mf: Vitamin World, Inc.	N/A	N/A	400[1]
B-6 (Pyridoxine)			
Akyma Pharmaceuticals Vitamin B-6 (Pyridoxine HCl) 50 mg (1 tablet/day) Dist: Akyma Pharmaceuticals LLC	N/A	N/A	N/A
Mason natural® Vitamin B Supplement B-6 100 mg (1 tablet/ day) Dist: Mason Vitamins, Inc.	N/A	N/A	N/A
Puritan's Pride® Vitamin B-6 100 mg (1 tablet/day)* Mf: Puritan's Pride, Inc.	N/A	N/A	N/A

B-5[d] (mg)	B-6[e] (mg)	B-12[f] (mcg)	Biotin (mg)	Folic acid (mcg)
N/A	N/A	N/A	N/A	N/A
N/A	N/A	N/A	N/A	N/A
N/A	50	N/A	N/A	N/A
N/A	100	N/A	N/A	N/A
N/A	100	N/A	N/A	N/A

continued

Product (label info.)	Labeled amount of B vitamins		
	B-1[a] (mg)	B-2[b] (mg)	B-3[c] (mg)
B-12 (Cyanocobalamin)			
Country Life® Hypoallergenic Vitamin B-12 500 mcg (1 tablet/ day) Mf: Country Life	N/A	N/A	N/A
Equaline™ High Potency 1000 mcg Vitamin B-12, Natural, Time Release (1 tablet/day) Dist: Albertsons, Inc.	N/A	N/A	N/A
Puritan's Pride® Sublingual B-12 Microlozenges 500 mcg (1 microlozenge/ day)* Mf: Puritan's Pride, Inc.	N/A	N/A	N/A
Puritan's Pride® Time Release Vitamin B-12 1000 mcg ENER-B® (1 tablet/ day)* Mf: Puritan's Pride, Inc.	N/A	N/A	N/A
Rexall® Sublingual High Potency B-12 2500 mcg (1 microlozenge/ day)* Mf: Rexall, Inc.	N/A	N/A	N/A

B-5[d] (mg)	B-6[e] (mg)	B-12[f] (mcg)	Biotin (mg)	Folic acid (mcg)
N/A	N/A	500	N/A	N/A
N/A	N/A	1000	N/A	N/A
N/A	N/A	500	N/A	N/A
N/A	N/A	1000	N/A	N/A
N/A	N/A	2500	N/A	N/A

continued

Product (label info.)	Labeled amount of B vitamins		
	B-1[a] (mg)	B-2[b] (mg)	B-3[c] (mg)
SISU Vitamin B-12 1000 mcg (1 capsule/day) Mf: SISU Inc.	N/A	N/A	N/A
Sundown® Benefits B-12 High Potency 1000 mcg (1 tablet/ day)* Mf: Sundown Inc.	N/A	N/A	N/A
Vitamin World® Naturally Inspired™ Sublingual B-12 Microlozenges 500 mcg (1 microlozenge/ day)* Mf: Vitamin World, Inc.	N/A	N/A	N/A
Vitamin World® Naturally Inspired™ Time Release Vitamin B-12 1000 mcg (1 tablet/ day)* Dist by Vitamin World, Inc.	N/A	N/A	N/A
Vitamin World® Naturally Inspired™ Sublingual Vitamin B-12 5000 mcg (1 lozenge/day)* Mf: Vitamin World, Inc	N/A	N/A	N/A

B-5[d] (mg)	B-6[e] (mg)	B-12[f] (mcg)	Biotin (mg)	Folic acid (mcg)
N/A	N/A	1000	N/A	N/A
N/A	N/A	1000	N/A	N/A
N/A	N/A	500	N/A	N/A
N/A	N/A	1000[1]	N/A	N/A
N/A	N/A	5000	N/A	N/A

continued

Product (label info.)	Labeled amount of B vitamins		
	B-1[a] (mg)	B-2[b] (mg)	B-3[c] (mg)
Biotin			
Nature's Bounty® High Potency Biotin 1000 mcg (1 tablet/day)* Mf: Nature's Bounty, Inc.	N/A	N/A	N/A
Nature's Life® Biotin 2,500 mcg (1 capsule/day) Dist: Nature's Life	N/A	N/A	N/A
Puritan's Pride® Super Biotin 5000 mcg (1 capsule/day)* Mf: Puritan's Pride, Inc.	N/A	N/A	N/A
Rexall® Extreme Biotin 1500 mcg (1 tablet/day)* Mf: Rexall, Inc.	N/A	N/A	N/A
Vitamin World® Naturally Inspired™ Super Biotin 5000 mcg (1 capsule/day)* Mf: Vitamin World, Inc.	N/A	N/A	N/A

B-5[d] (mg)	B-6[e] (mg)	B-12[f] (mcg)	Biotin (mg)	Folic acid (mcg)
N/A	N/A	N/A	1000	N/A
N/A	N/A	N/A	2500	N/A
N/A	N/A	N/A	5000	N/A
N/A	N/A	N/A	1500	N/A
N/A	N/A	N/A	5000	N/A

continued

Product (label info.)	Labeled amount of B vitamins		
	B-1[a] (mg)	B-2[b] (mg)	B-3[c] (mg)
Folic Acid			
Natural Factors® Folic Acid 1 mg, Plus 20 mg C (1 tablet/ day) Dist: Natural Factors	N/A	N/A	N/A
Puritan's Pride® Folic Acid 800 mcg (1 tablet/day)* Mf: Puritan's Pride, Inc.	N/A	N/A	N/A
🍁 Swiss™ Natural Sources Folic Acid 1 mg Plus, USP (1 tablet/day) Dist: Swiss Herbal Remedies Ltd.	N/A	N/A	N/A

‡ See also "More Brand Information," page 675.

[a] Thiamin

[b] Riboflavin

[c] Niacin

[d] Pantothenic acid

[e] Pyridoxine

[f] Cyanocobalin

N/A—Not applicable

🏃 Product passed optional Athletic Banned-Screening Program

[1] Maximum suggested serving size exceeds Upper Tolerable Intake Level (UL) for niacin for adults 19 and older.

🍁 Purchased from a retailer in Canada.

*Tested through CL's Voluntary Certification Program prior to, at time of, or after initial posting of the product review.

	B-5[d] (mg)	B-6[e] (mg)	B-12[f] (mcg)	Biotin (mg)	Folic acid (mcg)
	N/A	N/A	N/A	N/A	1000
	N/A	N/A	N/A	N/A	800
	N/A	N/A	N/A	N/A	1000

Chromium

An essential trace mineral that your body needs in small amounts, chromium is important for insulin function. Chromium picolinate may help some people with type 2 diabetes decrease fasting blood glucose levels as well as levels of insulin and glycosylated hemoglobin (HbA1c). Chromium may also produce modest weight loss, although the evidence is mixed. (See "Weight Loss Supplements: Bitter Orange, Green Tea, Hydroxycitric Acid, 7-Keto-DHEA, Pyruvate," page 202, volume 1, for other ingredients used for weight loss). Chromium may increase high-density lipoprotein (HDL) levels when these levels are lowered by use of beta-blockers.

Quality Concerns and Product Testing

Neither the FDA nor any other federal or state agency routinely tests supplements for quality prior to sale. Yet potential problems can exist with chromium supplements.

Amount of Key Ingredient: Knowing that a product contains the claimed ingredients and amounts is important. Too little chromium in the product may mean you do not get the expected effect and waste money. On the other hand, too much chromium can produce negative effects. In fact, some case reports indicate toxicity with chromium dosages over 600 mcg a day; rare reports show toxicity at dosages as low as over 200 mcg per day. Consequently, CL measured the amount of chromium in all products.

Hexavalent Chromium (Chromium VI) Contamination: Our bodies require trivalent chromium (chromium III); hexavalent chromium (chromium VI) is a somewhat toxic form of chromium that does not occur naturally in significant amounts but is formed as a by-product of the chemical and welding industries. Ingesting large amounts of hexavalent chromium can cause stomach upsets and ulcers, convulsions, kidney and liver damage, and even death. It is also a carcinogen and is the form of chromium implicated by consumer advocate Erin Brockovich as causing cancers in and around Hinkley, California (as depicted in the film *Erin Brockovich*). Although it should not be found in chromium supplements, it has occurred as a contaminant. Consequently, all of the chromium products were tested for levels of hexavalent chromium.

Lead: Lead is found as a contaminant in a small percentage of supplements, particularly those made with mineral or herbal ingredients. In fetuses, infants, and children, even low levels of lead can adversely affect neurobehavioral development and cognitive function. In adults, lead at somewhat higher levels can cause elevated blood pressure, anemia, and adversely affect the nervous and reproductive systems. Consequently, all of the products were tested for levels of lead.

Tablet Disintegration: Products that cannot properly disintegrate (break apart) may not fully deliver their ingredients. Consequently, all tablets and caplets were tested for their ability to disintegrate, or break apart, for proper release of their contents.

Caffeine: Caffeine is commonly found in weight-loss supplements, added directly or from herbal ingredients such as kola nut, green tea, guarana, and yerba maté. The total amount of caffeine in supplements is often not disclosed. Because of caffeine's potential side effects, it is useful to know the amount of caffeine in a daily dose. Consequently, caffeine levels were determined for any product labeled to contain caffeine or caffeine-containing herbs.

ConsumerLab.com purchased and tested six products. For more information on testing procedures, see the appropriate section in "ConsumerLab.com's Testing Methods and Standards," page 654.

Test Findings

Among the six products that ConsumerLab.com selected for testing, only three passed testing. Problems identified are noted by product.

EZ-Trim contained only 25% of its chromium—despite the fact that its label has a "cGMP certified" seal and indicates that it is "laboratory tested" and made with "pharmaceutical grade ingredients." It also contained 180 mg of caffeine per daily serving, equal to 4.5 cans of cola.

TRIMSPA X32 provided 42% *more* chromium than claimed, yielding 641 mcg of chromium per maximum daily serving. This is a high dose and is of concern because liver and kidney toxicity have been associated with long-term daily use of amounts over 600 mcg. This product also contained 346 mg of caffeine (equivalent to 8.6 cans of cola) in a maximum daily serving.

TRIMSPA X32 and Life Extension™ Chromium 200 mcg Caps were both found to contain relatively high levels of hexavalent chromium, a potential carcinogen and toxin. To pass the testing,

ConsumerLab.com required products to have no more than 0.1% of their total chromium in this form. In these two products, 0.4% and 3.8%, respectively, of the total chromium was hexavalent chromium. Whether these amounts are sufficient to cause harm is not known, but it seems prudent to avoid such exposure.

The other three chromium products passed testing and contained their claimed amounts of chromium and were free of contaminants. None of the products were contaminated with lead. All of the tablets and capsules broke apart properly.

Products that were selected for testing and a summary of the results are listed alphabetically in Test Results for Chromium Supplements. Also included in the list are other products (indicated with an asterisk) that have met the same criteria through CL's Voluntary Certification Program (see Selection and Testing, page 25, volume 1).

ConsumerTips™ for Buying and Using

Food Sources: Although the concentration of chromium in foods can vary widely from batch to batch, good food sources include organ meats, brewer's yeast, whole grains, cheese, prunes, nuts, asparagus, mushrooms, beer, coffee, tea, and wine. Estimates of chromium intake from diet in the U.S. are roughly 25 micrograms for women and 33 micrograms for men, amounts that are generally adequate to avoid severe deficiency but that may leave some people, such as women who are nursing, slightly deficient (see Adequate Intake). To get levels used therapeutically, however, supplements are generally needed.

Supplements: Various forms of chromium are available. Chromium picolinate and chromium polynicotinate are better absorbed than chromium chloride. Theoretical safety concerns have been raised about chromium picolinate, but none have been substantiated (see Concerns and Cautions). High-chromium yeast supplements are also available.

Some chromium product labels include the term *GTF*. GTF is not an ingredient but is a marketing term alluding to the outdated concept of "glucose tolerance factor." This concept is based on decades-old research, which concluded that the body combined chromium with nicotinate and other substances to form a large molecule named GTF. In turn, GTF was supposed to help control blood sugar. Certain foods, such as brewer's yeast, were thought to contain already formed GTF. For this reason, products containing chromium polynicotinate, or brewer's yeast extracts, sometimes use the term GTF in their labeling. However, current thinking is that GTF does not exist; instead, researchers think the substance was inadvertently produced by chemists themselves during their attempts to study the effects of chromium.

Current thinking also suggests that chromium influences blood sugar by combining with a small protein named "low molecular weight chromium-binding substance," or LMWCr (also called chromodulin). LMWCr does not contain nicotinate, and, like all proteins, if it were supplied by foods, it would be broken down in the digestive tract before being absorbed. Thus, the GTF labeling on chromium products most likely does not have any meaningful connotation.

In Diabetes: Taking 500 mcg twice daily significantly decreases HbA1c levels (a marker of blood sugar control) after two months of treatment, although taking 100 mcg twice daily can take up to 4 months to decrease these levels. High dose usage can be a concern, however (see Concerns and Cautions, page 356). Diabetics should check with their doctors before using chromium; if the supplement does improve blood sugar control, medication reduction may be necessary.

To Prevent Hypoglycemia: Taking 200 mg of chromium chloride daily for three months seems to improve symptoms and increase blood glucose levels in patients with reactive hypoglycemia.

Weight-Loss: Although its weight-loss benefits in healthy individuals have not been proven, dosage used in weight-loss studies ranged from 200 to 400 mcg of chromium daily. Dosages as low as 50 mcg have also been used.

Adequate Intake: Adequate Intakes (AI) have been established for chromium by the Food and Nutrition Board of the National Academy of Sciences and are as follows: 11 micrograms (mcg) for children ages 1 to 3, and 15 mcg for children ages 4 to 8. For boys ages 9 to 13, it is 25 mcg; for girls, it is 21 mcg. For males ages 14 to 50, it is 35 mcg. For females ages 14 to 18, it is 24 mcg, rising to 25 mcg for those ages 19 to 50. For men 51 years and older, it is 30 mcg; for women ages 51 and older it is 20 mcg. Women who are pregnant need 29 mcg if they are 18 years or younger and 30 mcg if 19 years and older. Lactating women need 44 mcg if they are 18 years or younger, and 45 mcg if they are 19 years or older.

UL: No Tolerable Upper Intake Level (UL) for chromium has been set because research regarding the long-term safety of chromium supplementation is lacking; however, it is thought that dosages less than 200 mcg per day are safe. Pregnant woman and nursing mothers should not take dosages above the AI described above.

Concerns and Cautions

Chromium is generally well tolerated. However, some patients can experience cognitive, perceptual, and motor dysfunction at doses as low as 200 to 400 mcg a day. Some patients also experience headaches, insomnia, sleep disturbances, irritability, and mood changes.

Although not common, significant adverse effects have been reported with chronic use of chromium picolinate. Doses of 600 to 2400 mcg a day have been associated with anemia, thrombocytopenia, hemolysis, hepatic dysfunction, and renal failure in some patients; however, it is not clear if chromium is responsible for these effects. One report indicates that the condition of a patient who had acute hepatitis and was taking only 200 mcg chromium polynicotinate daily for five months improved when the supplement was discontinued.

Acute chromium toxicity can cause vomiting, diarrhea, hemorrhage, and blood loss into the gastrointestinal tract resulting in cardiogenic shock.

Oral chromium supplements can cause allergic reactions in people with chromate or leather contact allergy.

Because picolinic acids might affect neurotransmitter levels, chromium picolinate should be used with caution in people with depression, bipolar disease, or psychosis.

One highly preliminary study suggests that chromium picolinate might damage DNA.

Test Results for Chromium Supplements

Product (label info: amount of chromium and dosing)‡ Daily: Mf suggested amount of chromium Manufacturer (Mf) or distributor (Dist)	Test Results			
	Approved or not approved	Contained labeled amount of key ingredient(s)	Acceptable levels of hexavalent chromium and lead**	Caffeine (mg)/ day
EZ-Trim™ (100 mcg/capsule, 4/day) Daily: 400 mcg Mf: Scientific Weight Loss Labs	*not* approved	Only 25% claimed chromium	✔	179 (equals 4.5 cans of cola)
Life Extension™ Chromium 200 mcg Caps[1] (200 mcg/capsule, 1/day) Daily: 200 mcg Dist: Life Extension Foundation Buyers Club, Inc.	*not* approved	✔	High level of hexavalent chromium (3.85%)	N/A
MegaFood® GTF Chromium (100 mcg/capsule, 1/day Daily: 100 mcg Mf: MegaFood®	approved	✔	✔	N/A

continued

Product (label info.)	Test Results			
	Approval	Contained labeled	Acceptable levels**	Caffeine (mg)/ day
New Chapter® GTF Chromium (200 mcg/capsule, 1/day) Daily: 200 mcg Mf/Dist: New Chapter Inc.	approved	✔	✔	N/A
Nutrilite® Chrompic Extra* (100 mcg/ capsule, 3/day) Daily: 300 mcg Dist: Access Business Group Inter-national LLC	approved	✔	✔	N/A
Thermosculpt™*** (100 mcg and 250 mg bitter orange extract/ softgel, 4/day) Daily: 400 mcg Dist: 4 Your Health	approved	✔	✔	None

Product (label info.)	Test Results			
	Approval	Contained labeled	Acceptable levels**	Caffeine (mg)/ day
TRIMSPA® X32 Original Formula[2] (75 mcg/tablet, 3–6/day) Daily: 255–450 mcg Dist: Trimspa	*not* approved	42% more chromium than claimed. (Use maximum dosage [641 mcg] with caution.)	High level of hexavalent chromium (0.4%)	173–346 (equals 4.3–8.6 cans of cola)

N/A—Not applicable: Disintegration test applies only to tablets and caplets. Not applicable to chewable products, powders, capsules, liquid, and time-release forms.

✔ Check indicates the results met the criteria listed in the column heading.

‡ See also "More Brand Information," page 675.

*Tested through CL's Voluntary Certification Program before, at the time of, or after the initial review.

**All mineral/botanical products tested for lead contamination. Percentage of chromium VI is %wt/wt of hexavalent chromium to total chromium.

***See also Bitter Orange, page 212, volume 1.

[1] Life Extension (LE) has contacted CL asserting that this product is not contaminated with amount of hexavalent chromium stated above. LE alleges that the EPA testing method used by CL "creates" the hexavalent form. However, LE has not provided product test results to support these claims. In addition, other chromium products tested by CL made with the same brand of chromium in the LE product were not found to contain the relatively high amount of hexavalent chromium in the LE product. CL remains open to evaluating additional information regarding this matter.

[2] The distributor of TRIMSPA X32 claims that, according to its own testing, the product meets its label claims and is not contaminated. CL remains confident in the results presented above.

Iron

Iron is an essential mineral that the body requires in small amounts. It is widely available in foods including meat, poultry, and fish as well as dried fruits, grains, and green leafy vegetables. Iron from plant sources is absorbed half as well as that from animal sources. The average diet provides about 10 to 20 milligrams (mg) of iron a day.

Iron is needed to manufacture hemoglobin, which enables red blood cells to transfer oxygen to the body's tissues. Severe or prolonged iron deficiency is the leading cause of anemia in the United States, affecting about 5% of women and 2% of men.

Symptoms of anemia include easy fatigability, shortness of breath with mild exercise, and lethargy. Some evidence suggests that even mild iron deficiency, too mild to cause anemia, may cause fatigue and impair sports performance.

Iron deficiency is most common in menstruating women but also is commonly seen in children and pregnant women. Low iron levels also may result from excessive bleeding, burns, and hemodialysis as well as stomach and intestinal problems. Drugs that reduce stomach acid may also impair iron absorption.

During pregnancy, iron deficiency can result in preterm delivery and low-birth-weight babies. Among children, iron deficiency is most common from ages 6 to 24 months, where it can cause developmental and behavioral problems. If iron deficiency is extremely severe, some of these problems can be irreversible.

At the other end of the spectrum, too much iron can be toxic and is a leading cause of poisoning in children, which is why supplements with iron must be sold in childproof containers. In addition, some evidence hints that mildly excessive iron intake could increase risk of heart disease, cancer and type 2 diabetes. See Concerns and Cautions (page 363) for other risks of excessive iron intake.

In addition, iron supplements have shown some promise for reducing the dry cough caused by drugs in the angiotensin-converting enzyme inhibitor family (ACE inhibitors).

How much iron should a supplement contain? The recommended daily intake for iron for individuals without special needs ranges from 7 mg to 27 mg a day, depending on gender and stage of life. But people's diets vary; hence, the amount of supplementation necessary varies. Consequently, the amount of iron in supplements varies widely among brands. Moreover, iron is available in many forms. All can supply adequate iron, although some may be better tolerated than others. (See ConsumerTips™ for Buying and Using, page 362, for information about forms of iron in supplements.)

Quality Concerns and Product Testing

In ConsumerLab.com's previous testing of iron supplements in 2001, one product failed for containing too much lead and another failed for containing less than three-quarters of its claimed amount of iron. In addition, lead is a potentially harmful contaminant found in some mineral and herbal supplements. In 1997, the U.S. Food and Drug Administration (FDA) reported that several iron-containing supplements had been recalled because of excessive levels of lead.

Because no government agency is responsible for routinely testing iron supplements for their contents or quality, ConsumerLab. com independently evaluated iron products to determine whether they contained the iron stated on their labels. The products also were tested for contamination with lead. Iron tablets and caplets that were not chewable or time-release were additionally tested for their ability to break apart, or disintegrate, as needed for absorption. (See the appropriate section in "ConsumerLab.com's Testing Methods and Standards," page 655, for more information.)

Test Findings

ConsumerLab.com purchased 16 iron supplements, several of which included other nutrients, such as vitamin C, folic acid and other B vitamins, and various herbs. Of these 16 products, all passed the testing—an improvement over results from 2001. They contained what they claimed, disintegrated properly, and lacked lead contamination.

Some products will be more appropriate for you than others depending on your particular needs. The products vary by dose, type of iron, and form (that is, chewable tablet, time-release tablet, liquid, and so forth) and some contain additional ingredients.

The 11 products that were selected for testing and a summary of the results are listed alphabetically in Test Results for Iron Supplements. Also included in the list are 5 other products (indicated with an asterisk) that met the same criteria through CL's Voluntary Certification Program (see Selection and Testing, page 25, volume 1).

Many of the products may have been designed for treating iron deficiency and, therefore, exceed the Recommended Dietary Allowance (RDA) as well as the upper level (UL) of tolerable intake for iron. Under a physician's supervision, it's acceptable to exceed the limits because the potential consequences of untreated deficiency may be more severe than the potential adverse effects of a high intake.

ConsumerTips™ for Buying and Using

To Treat Anemia: For individuals diagnosed with iron-deficiency anemia, the recommended dose depends on the severity of the anemia and weight of the individual. Your physician should determine the dose.

In general, a typical adult dosage for correcting anemia is 100 to 200 mg daily, divided into two or three doses. About two months is usually required to restore hemoglobin levels. Many more months of iron supplementation may be required to fully build up iron stores.

To Prevent Anemia: The daily recommended intake of iron for healthy individuals depends on your gender and life stage. The FDA requires that dietary supplements state on their labels the % Daily Value for certain vitamins and minerals. However, the percentages given may not reflect the latest recommendations. Moreover, the labels are unlikely to provide information indicating whether the ingredients exceed upper tolerable intake levels (UL), as many do, because the FDA doesn't require that information.

The following information will help you determine which amounts are appropriate for your gender and life stage. When reading labels, remember that 1,000 mcg (micrograms) equals 1 mg (milligram) and that 1,000 mg equals 1 gram.

Recommended intake: The RDA (Recommended Daily Allowance) for iron is 7 mg for children ages 1 to 3 and 10 mg for children ages 4 to 8. It then decreases to 8 mg for children ages 9 to 13. For males ages 14 to 18, the RDA is 11 mg; 19 and older, it decreases to 8 mg. For females, ages 14 to 18, the RDA is 15 mg; 19 to 50, it's 18 mg, decreasing to 8 mg ages 51 and older.

Because of fetal needs, the RDA for pregnant women is to 27 mg. For breast-feeding women younger than age 18, the RDA is 10 mg; for ages 19 and older, it's 9 mg. Also, postmenopausal women taking hormone replacement therapy should consume more iron because the therapy can cause periodic uterine bleeding. Oral contraceptives may reduce menstrual blood loss, so women taking them may need less daily iron.

Upper limit: High daily amounts of iron can cause gastrointestinal distress, especially when iron supplements are consumed on an empty stomach. The UL is 40 mg for children younger than age 13 and 45 mg for everyone else. However, these limits may be too high for people with hereditary hemochromatosis, who are at unique risk for accumulating harmful levels of iron.

Forms of Iron: Several different forms of iron are used in supplements. The actual amount of usable "elemental" iron per milligram of iron compound varies depending on the form, but fortunately, the consumer doesn't need to do calculations; the manufacturer does this. The usable amount is what appears on the label.

Generally, the least expensive forms of iron are ferrous sulfate, ferrous fumarate, and ferrous gluconate. If you have trouble tolerating these forms of iron because of gastrointestinal discomfort, consider chelated iron, time-release iron supplements, ferrous bisglycinate, or ferrous glycinate. All of them are fairly expensive but may be the least likely to cause stomach upset. Another form, carbonyl iron, may present a reduced risk of harm in an accidental overdose. Carbonyl iron, consequently, is the ingredient many children's supplements contain and may be preferred by parents of small children. However, carbonyl iron requires adequate stomach acid for absorption. Therefore, it should be taken with food and not used with medications that reduce stomach acid. Injectable iron also is available under the supervision of a health professional.

Still another way to deal with gastric upset is to take an iron supplement with food. Though combining the supplement with food may decrease iron absorption, taking it with a vitamin C–rich food may offset that effect because vitamin C boosts iron absorption. In fact, some iron supplements contain vitamin C as an added ingredient to aid absorption.

Remember that many antacids can decrease iron absorption, as can soy protein, coffee, tea, eggs, whole-grain cereals and breads, and spinach. Iron absorption also can be reduced by high doses of calcium, zinc, manganese, magnesium, or copper. When consuming one of these foods or high-dose mineral supplements, wait one to two hours to take your iron supplement.

Concerns and Cautions

Although iron supplements are safe and potentially helpful when taken correctly, excessive iron intake can be harmful.

The most common immediate side effect of iron supplements is gastrointestinal distress, a symptom that often occurs when a high-dose iron supplement is taken on an empty stomach.

Other problems can occur with prolonged excessive intake of iron. For example, although pregnant women are generally encouraged to take iron supplements, supplementation beyond the recommended amount may *increase* complications of pregnancy. Also one study found that non-iron-deficient, breast-fed infants do not benefit from iron supplements. These infants might even experience an overall decrease in health if given iron supplementation.

Furthermore, observational studies have found associations between mildly excessive levels of stored iron in the body and heart disease, cancer, and type 2 diabetes. This does not prove that excessive iron intake causes those diseases, but it does suggest a connection. On this basis, CL suggests that people should not take iron supplements unless blood tests have shown them to be iron deficient. Note that nonvegetarian adult men and postmenopausal women are unlikely to lack adequate iron.

Iron at greatly excessive doses taken continually can result in toxicity, causing cirrhosis, coronary heart disease, congestive heart failure, and other problems. Also, vitamin C increases iron absorption. People who take very high doses of vitamin C (a gram or more daily) are at increased risk of iron toxicity. Toxicity is of particular concern for individuals with hemochromatosis, a genetic condition affecting 1 out of 200 to 500 people. With hemochromatosis, excessive amounts of iron build up in the body's tissues and organs.

Iron supplements also may reduce the absorption of certain drugs such as levodopa, levothyroxine, penicillamine, quinolone antibiotics, and tetracycline antibiotics. Some of these drugs may, conversely, interfere with iron absorption.

Remember, iron supplements are a leading cause of poisoning in children younger than age 6. Just a few adult tablets can cause serious poisoning, so keep iron products away from children's reach. To help reduce the number of such poisonings, supplements containing more than 30 mg of iron (other than carbonyl iron) can be sold only in child-resistant bottles or in single-dose packaging.

Test Results for Iron Supplements

Product (label info: elemental iron/ unit, form of iron, dosing)‡ Manufacturer (Mf) or Distributor (Dist)	Test Results			
	Approved or not approved	Iron content met claim	Acceptable level of lead	Broke apart
Douglas Laboratories® Timed Release Iron (27 mg/time-release tablet, *iron carbonyl*, 2 tablets/day**) Mf: Douglas Laboratories	approved**	✔	✔	N/A
Feosol® Ferrous Sulfate Iron Supplement Therapy, (65 mg/tablet, *ferrous sulfate*, 1 tablet/day**) Dist: GlaxoSmithKline	approved**	✔	✔	✔
Fergon® Ferrous Gluconate High Potency Iron Supplement (27 mg/tablet, ferrous gluconate, 1 tablet/ day) Dist: Bayer Healthcare LLC	approved	✔	✔	✔

continued

Product (label info.)	Test Results			
	Approval	**Met claim**	**Acceptable level**	**Broke apart**
Floradix® Iron+Herbs Liquid Extract Formula Dietary Supplement, (5 mg/ teaspoon, *ferrous gluconate,* 4 teaspoons/ day) Mf: Salus-Haus (Product of Germany)	approved	✔	✔	N/A
Good Neighbor Pharmacy® Iron Tablets (Ferrous Sulfate) Iron Supplement Therapy, (65 mg/tablet, *ferrous sulfate,* 1 tablet/day**) Dist: Bergen Brunswig Drug Company	approved**	✔	✔	✔
Natrol™ Liquid Iron Supplement with Vitamins, Herbs and Tropical Fruit Extracts, (3.6 mg/ teaspoon, *amino acid chelate,* 4 teaspoons/ day) Dist: Natrol Inc	approved	✔	✔	N/A

Product (label info.)	Test Results			
	Approval	Met claim	Acceptable level	Broke apart
Nature's Plus® The Energy Supplements® High Potency Chewable Iron with Vitamin C and Herbs, (27 mg/chewable tablet, *amino acid chelate*, 1 tablet/day) Dist: Nature's Plus	approved	✔	✔	N/A
Nutrilite® Tri-Iron Folic, (10 mg/tablet, *ferrous bisglycinate, ferrous fumarate,* 1-3 tablets/day)* Dist:Access Business Group International LLC	approved	✔	✔	✔
NEWtritional Defense™ Naturally Blackstrap Iron Chelated Supplement, (27 mg/tablet, *ferrous gluconate,* 1 tablet/day) Dist: Marlyn Nutraceuticals Inc	approved	✔	✔	✔
Puritan's Pride® Easy Iron, Iron Glycinate, (28 mg/capsule *ferrous bisglycinate,* 1 capsule/day)* Mf: Puritan's Pride Inc	approved	✔	✔	N/A

continued

Product (label info.)	Test Results			
	Approval	Met claim	Acceptable level	Broke apart
Puritan's Pride® Ferrous Gluconate* (28 mg/tablet, *ferrous gluconate,* 1 tablet/day) Mf: Puritan's Pride Inc	approved	✔	✔	✔
Rite Aid High Potency Iron, (27 mg/tablet, *ferrous sulfate,* 1 tablet/day) Dist: Rite Aid Corporation	approved	✔	✔	✔
Safeway Select™ Premium Quality High Potency Iron, (27 mg/ tablet, *ferrous sulfate,* 1 tablet/day) Dist: Safeway Inc	approved	✔	✔	✔
SLOWFE® Slow Release Iron + Folic Acid, (47.5 mg/time-release tablet, *ferrous sulfate,* 1-2 tablets/ day**) Dist: Novartis Consumer Health Inc	approved**	✔	✔	N/A
Sundown Benefits® Carbonyl Iron, (50 mg/tablet, *carbonyl iron,* 2 tablets/day**)* Dist: Rexall Sundown Inc	approved**	✔	✔	✔

Product (label info.)	Test Results			
	Approval	**Met claim**	**Acceptable level**	**Broke apart**
Vitamin World® Naturally Inspired™ Easy Iron, Iron Glycinate, (28 mg/ capsule, *ferrous bisglycinate,* 1 capsule/day)* Mf: Vitamin World Inc	approved	✔	✔	N/A

*Tested through CL's Voluntary Certification Program

N/A—Not applicable: Disintegration test applies to tablets and caplets.

✔ Check indicates the results met the criteria listed in the column heading.

‡ See also "More Brand Information," page 675.

**Suggested maximum daily dose exceeds UL; for treating iron deficiency.

Magnesium

Magnesium is an essential mineral for the body and as many as 15% of adults in the United States may take a supplement containing magnesium. In addition to magnesium-only supplements, supplemental magnesium can be obtained from laxatives, antacids, multivitamin and multimineral products and calcium supplements containing magnesium. Magnesium comes in a variety of chemical forms, including magnesium oxide, magnesium gluconate, and magnesium citrate. (For more information, see ConsumerTips™ for Buying and Using, "Bone-Health Supplements: Calcium and Vitamin D," page 31, volume 1, and "Multivitamin/Multimineral Supplements," page 380.)

Magnesium is needed for proper metabolism and nervous system functioning. Although sufficient magnesium can be obtained easily from your diet, magnesium deficiency may affect a small percentage of the population in whom it may modestly elevate blood pressure and increase the risk of osteoporosis. Conditions that may deplete magnesium include alcohol abuse, diabetes, diseases of the digestive tract, such as ulcerative colitis, Crohn's disease and celiac sprue, and use of medications such as cisplatin and certain diuretics. Severe magnesium deficiency causes irritability, muscle weakness, and irregular heartbeat, but deficiency sufficient to cause these symptoms is rare.

Use of magnesium supplements may help prevent a number of conditions including hearing loss from excessive noise, migraine headaches (including menstrual migraines), menstrual pain, and PMS.

Despite some claims to the opposite, some evidence suggests that oral magnesium supplements do not help prevent the heart irregularity called atrial fibrillation nor help prevent kidney stones. Intravenous magnesium, rather than oral magnesium supplements, is sometimes used in hospitals to treat acute asthma, overdoses of certain drugs, osmotic coma, diabetic ketoacidosis, pancreatitis, hyperthyroidism, hepatitis, and other conditions.

Quality Concerns and Product Testing

Like other supplements, neither the FDA nor any other federal or state agency routinely tests magnesium products for quality. However, quality issues for magnesium supplements can include the following:

Labeled Amount: Does the product really contain the labeled amount of magnesium? Too little magnesium in a supplement is a problem if relying on it to prevent or correct a deficiency. Excessive consumption of oral magnesium frequently causes diarrhea. Although an individual with healthy kidneys is unlikely to be able to take enough magnesium orally to elevate blood levels, if excessive levels do occur, potentially dangerous heart and nerve-related symptoms may develop. Individuals with severe kidney disease should not take magnesium supplements.

Purity: Many sources of magnesium, like other minerals, may naturally contain amounts of heavy metals such as lead. In children, fetuses, and infants, even low levels of lead can adversely affect neurobehavioral development and cognitive function. In adults, lead at somewhat higher levels can cause elevated blood pressure and anemia, and adversely affect the nervous and reproductive systems. Lead is of particular concern during pregnancy as the mother can transfer it to the fetus.

Availability: Once in your body, will the pill break down properly so that it can be absorbed?

Side Effects at Suggested Dosage: ConsumerLab. com reviewed the levels of magnesium to determine if any product provided doses high enough so as to carry a risk of adverse side effects. Those that exceeded upper tolerable limits are footnoted.

ConsumerLab.com, as part of its mission to independently evaluate products that affect health, wellness, and nutrition, purchased many leading magnesium supplements products sold in the U.S. and tested them to determine whether they 1) possessed the claimed amount of magnesium, 2) could disintegrate properly in order to be available for absorption, and 3) were free of unacceptable levels of lead (see the appropriate section in "ConsumerLab.com's Testing Methods and Standards," page 656.)

Test Findings

All of the products contained their claimed amounts of magnesium, and all tablets and caplets disintegrated properly when tested. However, the following two products contained much higher levels of lead than the others—more lead than allowed without a warning label in California.

Jamieson™, Natural Sources Calcium Magnesium contained 1.9 mcg of lead per daily serving, and Weil™, Andrew Weil,

M.D., Balanced Cal-Mag contained 2.3 mcg of lead per daily serving.

Although the FDA acknowledges the dangers of lead exposure, it has not set limits on the amount of lead in dietary supplements, nor has any state other than California. California requires a warning label on any supplement containing more than 0.5 micrograms (mcg) of lead per daily serving for a magnesium-only supplement or 1.5 micrograms of lead for supplements that also contain one gram of calcium, such as these two products. Although not dangerous in and of themselves, these products significantly and unnecessarily contribute to lead exposure. It is advisable to get as little lead as possible, particularly for fetuses and children because low amounts can affect their mental functioning.

The 15 products that were selected for testing and a summary of the results are listed alphabetically in Test Results for Magnesium Supplements. Also included in the list are six other products (indicated with an asterisk) that have met the same criteria through CL's Voluntary Certification Program (see Selection and Testing, page 25, volume 1).

ConsumerTips™ for Buying and Using

When buying magnesium, keep in mind the following information: In the products evaluated, the labeled amount of magnesium ranged from 30 milligrams to 500 milligrams a tablet. These amounts should be considered when comparing the costs of products. Product labels should indicate the amount of actual magnesium (or "elemental" magnesium) per dosage unit. This dosage information is important because magnesium actually makes up less than half of the weight of magnesium compounds. For example, the amount of magnesium in magnesium gluconate is only 5.8%, and it is 12% in magnesium chloride hexahydrate, 16.2% in magnesium citrate, 50% in magnesium glycinate, and 60.3% in magnesium oxide.

Nearly all of forms of magnesium can act as laxatives; magnesium hydroxide (milk of magnesia) is widely marketed for this purpose. Magnesium hydroxide and magnesium oxide are also used in antacid products. All these forms, as well as magnesium chloride and others, are used in magnesium supplements. The sulfate form may also be used intravenously under medical supervision for seizures, uterine tetany, and other acute conditions.

Although all forms of magnesium are absorbed fairly well, absorption may vary. Magnesium oxide is thought to be less well absorbed than magnesium citrate; magnesium L-lactate dihydrate may be the most absorbable form of magnesium.

Products that contain calcium in addition to magnesium are sometimes touted as improving the absorption of these minerals or to make up for decreased absorption of one because of the other. However, in a healthy individual, the two minerals (at moderate doses) do not appear to interact or interfere with each other, and taking extra calcium is not necessary when supplementing with magnesium, nor vice versa. Nor is a specific ratio of the two minerals known to produce superior absorption. However, people at high risk for magnesium deficiency should consider taking calcium at bedtime to avoid inhibiting dietary magnesium absorption.

Your daily requirement for magnesium can be obtained through food sources without much difficulty, and generally speaking, the great majority of individuals in developed countries have an adequate intake. Especially rich sources of magnesium include whole grains, nuts, beans, avocado, shellfish, green leafy vegetables, coffee, tea and chocolate. A cup of whole-grain flour has nearly 200 mg of magnesium. A cupful of spinach or most beans, nuts, seeds, or trail mix offers anywhere from 50 mg to 150 mg of magnesium. A cup of milk, orange juice, or grapefruit juice provides about 80 mg.

The recommended daily allowance (RDA) for magnesium is 80 mg for children ages 1 to 3, 130 mg for those 4 to 8, and 240 mg for those 9 to 13. For males ages 14 to 18, it is 410 mg; for those 19 to 30, it falls to 400 mg, and for those ages 31 and older it is 420 mg. For females ages 14 to 18, it is 360 mg; for those 19 to 30, it falls to 310 mg, and for those ages 31 and older it is 320 mg. However, for pregnant women, it is 400 mg if 18 years or younger, 350 mg if 19 to 30, and 360 mg if 31 or older. For lactating women, it is 360 mg if 18 years or younger, 310 mg if 19 to 30, and 320 mg if 31 or older.

Bear in mind that the recommended amounts noted above are for total daily magnesium intake. The average daily intake of magnesium from food sources in the United States is approximately 320 mg; thus supplementation is likely to increase magnesium intake above nutritional needs.

When used as a treatment, magnesium is often recommended at doses of 250 to 600 mg daily.

Magnesium specifically from supplements can often cause diarrhea, which is why it is an ingredient in many laxatives. Diarrhea is particularly common in products also containing aluminum. However, taking magnesium with food can reduce the occurrence of diarrhea. Excessive magnesium levels in the blood can cause dangerous side effects, but oral supplements seldom actually raise blood levels in individuals with healthy kidneys. Tolerable Upper Intake Levels (UL) have been established for magnesium supplement intake. The UL is defined as "a level of chronic daily intake judged to be likely to pose no risk of adverse health effects to the most sensitive members of the healthy population." The UL recommendations (which apply specifically to magnesium consumed from supplements or other medications) are 65 mg for children ages 1 to 3, and 110 mg for those 4 to 8. For individuals ages 9 and older, the UL is 350 mg. Note that the UL for supplements sometimes are actually lower than the respective RDA, because side effects are not likely to occur from magnesium obtained from solely from foods.

Contrary to some reports, calcium and magnesium do not seem to affect each other's absorption in any significant way. Both calcium and magnesium are macrominerals; that is, their RDA are relatively high compared to microminerals such as zinc, for which only a few milligrams or microgram amounts are needed. However, because both magnesium and calcium supplements can interfere with the absorption of microminerals, your best bet is to take such minerals at a different time of day from a calcium or magnesium supplement. Because of the bulk of both magnesium and calcium, they are generally not found in multivitamin-multimineral products in doses equivalent to their RDA and are often sold separately or combined.

Concerns and Cautions

Individuals with kidney disease cannot properly control levels of electrolytes in the body; for this reason, taking magnesium (or any other mineral) can be very dangerous. People with severe heart disease or diseases of the intestines as well may have risks as well.

Magnesium interferes with the absorption of medications in the tetracycline family and can also interfere with the effectiveness of cellulose sodium phosphate and sodium polystyrene sulfonate.

Test Results for Magnesium Supplements

Product (label info: form of magnesium, amount of elemental magnesium/ unit, dosing)‡ Manufacturer (Mf) or Distributor (Dist)	Test Results		
	Approved or not approved	Contained labeled amount of magnesium	Acceptable level of lead
Magnesium			
Floradix® Magnesium Liquid Mineral Supplement (elemental magnesium, 250 mg/capful [20 mL], 1/day) Mf: Salus-Haus	approved	✔	✔
KAL® Magnesium Glycinate 400 (magnesium glycinate, 200 mg/tablet, 2/day) Mf: Nutraceutical Corp. for Makers of Kal, Inc.	approved[1]	✔	✔
Life Extension™ Magnesium (Citrate) 160 mg (magnesium citrate, 160 mg/capsule, 1–8/day) Dist: Life Extension Foundation Buyers Club Inc.	approved[1]	✔	✔
Longs® Natural Magnesium 250 mg, Product Benefit (magnesium oxide, 250 mg/ tablet, 1/day) Dist: Longs Drugs	approved	✔	✔

continued

Product (label info.)	Test Results		
	Approval	Contained labeled	Acceptable level
Nature Made Magnesium 250 mg (magnesium oxide, 250 mg/tablet, 1/day)* Dist: Nature Made Nutritional Products	approved	✔	✔
Nature's Bounty® High Potency Magnesium 500 mg (magnesium oxide, 500 mg/ tablet, 1/day)* Mf: Nature's Bounty, Inc.	approved[1]	✔	✔
NOW® Magnesium Caps (magnesium oxide, citrate and aspartate, 400 mg/ tablet, 1/day) Mf: NOW Foods	approved[1]	✔	✔
Puritan's Pride® Chelated Magnesium 30 mg (magnesium gluconate, 30 mg/tablet, 1/day)* Mf: Puritan's Pride, Inc.	approved	✔	✔
Rexall® Super Magnesium Oxide 250 mg (magnesium oxide, 250 mg/caplet, 1/day)* Mf: Rexall, Inc.	approved	✔	✔
Safeway Select™ Bones and Joints Minerals Magnesium 250 mg (magnesium oxide, 250 mg/tablet, 1/day) Dist: Safeway Inc.	approved	✔	✔

Product (label info.)	Test Results		
	Approval	Contained labeled	Acceptable level
Sundown® Essential Magnesium 250 mg (magnesium oxide, 250 mg/ caplet, 1/day)* Mf: Sundown, Inc.	approved	✔	✔
Vitamin World® Naturally Inspired™ Magnesium Citrate (magnesium citrate, 100 mg/tablet, 1/day)* Mf: Vitamin World, Inc.	approved[1]	✔	✔
Walgreen's® Magnesium 250 mg (magnesium oxide, 250 mg/tablet, 1/day) Dist: Walgreen's Co.	approved	✔	✔
Whole Foods™ Chelated Magnesium 200 mg (magnesium amino acid chelate and magnesium oxide, 200 mg/tablet, 1–3/day) Dist: Whole Foods Markets	approved	✔	✔
Magnesium with Calcium			
Jamieson™, Natural Sources Calcium Magnesium (magnesium oxide, 167 mg/ caplet, 3/day) Mf: Jamieson Laboratories	***not* approved[1]**	✔	Contained 1.9 mcg of lead per daily serving

continued

Product (label info.)	Test Results		
	Approval	**Contained labeled**	**Acceptable level**
Liquid Calcium Magnesium original formula, NF Formulas, Vanilla Flavor 1:1 Ca/Mg Ratio (magnesium oxide and citrate, 250 mg/ tablet, 2/day) Dist: Integrative Therapeutics Inc.	approved	✔	✔
Natural Factors® Calcium and Magnesium Citrate with D, plus potassium and zinc (magnesium oxide and citrate, 250 mg/tablet 2/day) Mf: Natural Factors, Canada, Dist: Natural Factors USA	approved[1]	✔	✔
Schiff Bone Care®, Calcium-Magnesium with vitamin D (magnesium oxide, 133 mg/ softgel, 3/day) Dist: Schiff Products	approved[1]	✔	✔
Slow-Mag® Tablets, Magnesium Chloride with Calcium (magnesium chloride hexahydrate, 64 mg/enteric coated tablet, 2/day) Dist: Purdue Products L.P.	approved	✔	✔
Source Naturals® Magnesium Chelate 100 mg (magnesium chelate, 100 mg/tablet, 1–4/day) Dist: Source Naturals, Inc.	approved[1]	✔	✔

Product (label info.)	Test Results		
	Approval	Contained labeled	Acceptable level
Weil™, Andrew Weil, M.D. Balanced Cal-Mag (magnesium chelate and magnesium citrate, 125 mg/ tablet, 4/day) Dist: Weil Nutritional Supplements	*not* approved	✔	2.3 mcg of lead/daily serving

✔ Check indicates the results met the criteria listed in the column heading.

‡ See also "More Brand Information," page 675.

*Tested through CL's Voluntary Certification Program before, at the time of, or after the initial review.

[1]Maximum suggested serving size exceeds Upper Tolerable Intake Level (UL) for magnesium (350 mg/day) for adults when taken within range of recommended daily servings and should be used with awareness of potential side effects, particularly diarrhea.

Multivitamin/Multimineral Supplements

Background

Multivitamins/multiminerals, referred to as "multis," are America's most popular dietary supplements. The ingredients vary widely by brand. There are no established standards on what multis should contain.

One reason for not having uniform standards is that people's diets and needs differ. Nutrient requirements and cautions vary, depending on age, gender, health status, use of substances such as alcohol or tobacco, and medications taken.

A major update of the recommendations for daily nutrient intake was issued by the Institute of Medicine in 2001. These are provided in this report in the ConsumerTips™ for Buying and Using, page 384. However, the U.S. Food and Drug Administration (FDA) has yet to require product labeling to include much of this new information in the % Daily Value (DV) listing that appears in the Supplement Facts panel on supplements. The current DVs are largely based on nutritional recommendations dating from 1968.

Products also can remain on store shelves for months or even years before being replaced with newer versions. Consequently, even if a manufacturer has reformulated its product to meet new recommendations, consumers may still be buying the older version.

In addition to selecting a product that appears to have the right ingredients, one should be confident that it contains what it claims, breaks down properly once in the body so its ingredients can be effectively utilized, and is free of impurities. Neither the U.S. government nor any agency is responsible for routinely testing multis or other dietary supplements for their contents or quality.

ConsumerLab.com, as part of its mission to independently evaluate products that affect health and nutrition, purchased many of the leading multivitamin/multimineral products sold in the U.S. and Canada, tested them for quality, and evaluated them against the most recently recommended Dietary Reference Intakes (DRIs).

Quality Concerns and Product Testing

Multivitamins/multiminerals are among those supplements most likely to have quality problems. They contain multiple ingredients and, therefore, more possibility of error. Earlier tests by ConsumerLab.com have found multis that were short on ingredients, failed to dissolve properly, or were contaminated with heavy metals.

ConsumerLab.com tested products for their amounts of several common labeled ingredients—folic acid, calcium, and vitamin A (retinol and beta-carotene)—as indicators of product quality. Not all the products were labeled to contain every one of these ingredients. Therefore, some were alternatively tested for other ingredients, such as vitamin C (ascorbic acid) in the absence of folic acid, and iron or zinc if calcium was not present (see "ConsumerLab.com's Testing Methods and Standards," page 657).

Products also were tested to determine if they disintegrated properly in order to dissolve and be absorbed in the body, and did not contain excessive and/or potentially harmful levels of lead, a contaminant of some mineral- and herbal-based products.

Products had to pass testing on all these criteria to be considered approved. In addition, ConsumerLab.com reviewed the levels of vitamins and minerals to determine if any product provided doses high enough to carry a risk of adverse side effects. Those that exceeded upper tolerable limits (ULs—see discussion that follows) are marked as such.

Test Findings

Among 21 products for adults and children that ConsumerLab.com independently selected and tested, only 10 met their claims and other quality standards. Two pet multivitamins were also tested, only one of which passed testing. The reasons that products failed are indicated in the table and described here by category of multivitamin/multimineral supplement.

General (Adult): Eniva® VIBE™, a liquid sold in packets, had only 54% of its claimed 5,000 IU of vitamin A. Healthy Moments™ Mint Cream Flavor Vitamin Strips contained none of its claimed vitamin A. It also contained 180% of its claimed 2 mg of niacin per strip. Swanson® Daily Multi-Vitamin & Mineral had only 77.5% of its claimed 400 mcg of folate per capsule. The Greatest Vitamin in the World had only 85% of its claimed 800 mcg of folate in its suggested nine capsules per day—although this still meets the adult RDA.

WEIL™ Andrew Weil, M.D. Daily Multivitamin for Optimum Health had only 73% of its claimed 10,000 IU of vitamin A (as beta-carotene) per tablet—although this still meets the adult RDA. It also had 251% of its claimed 60 mg of calcium—possibly an oversight of the calcium contributed by di-calcium phosphate, a binding agent listed among its inactive ingredients.

Women's: Nature's Plus® Especially Yours® Women's Multi-Vitamin failed to break apart properly, requiring more than one hour to disintegrate rather than the 30-minute limit established by the U.S. Pharmacopeia (USP). Such products may pass through the body without being fully utilized. It also contained 292% of its claimed 50 mg/tablet of calcium—possibly due to an oversight of the calcium contributed by the di-calcium phosphate in the product. The Vitamin Shoppe® Multivitamins Especially for Women was contaminated with 15.3 micrograms of lead per daily serving. This is more than ten times the amount of lead permitted without a warning label in California—the only state to regulate lead in supplements—and several times the normal daily exposure to lead. Lead at this level may not in itself be toxic to adults, but lead is stored in the body and unnecessary exposure should be avoided. This product should not be shared with children, as they are susceptible to lead poisoning at levels as low as 6 micrograms per day. This product also contained only 54% of its claimed 200 mg of calcium in its suggested daily dose of two tablets. *Update: Vitamin Shoppe* (January 23, 2007) issued a news release stating that it voluntarily removed the product from sale. It falsely suggested CL has hampered it in retesting its product. To the contrary, within three hours of being contacted by the company, CL furnished a two-page report with test results, methods (which were already available online), the product lot number, and additional information. Receipt was confirmed by Vitamin Shoppe vice president for Scientific and Regulatory Affairs. CL reiterated its policy permitting retesting by a third party. Vitamin Shoppe has not responded to this offer, nor published any information that refutes our findings.

Men's: Now® Adam™ Superior Men's Multi failed to break apart properly, taking 40 minutes to disintegrate rather than the 30 minutes set by the USP. Win™ Fuel Men's Formula had only 81% of its claimed 4,000 IU of vitamin (although this is still above the RDA of 3,000 IU for men) and only 75% of its claimed 400 mcg of folate.

Seniors: AARP Maturity Formula failed to break apart properly, taking 50 minutes to disintegrate rather than the 30 minutes set by the USP. *Update:* AARP (January 19, 2007) voluntarily withdrew the product from the market and is investigating the problem.

Children's: Hero Nutritionals™ Yummi® Bears contained 216% of its labeled amount of vitamin A, potentially delivering amounts in excess of those tolerable in children up to eight years old. The product contained 5,400 IU of vitamin A in the retinol form in a daily serving of three bears. The upper tolerable level (UL) set by the Institute of Medicine is 2,000 IU for children one to three years of age and 3,000 IU for those four to eight years old. Children of these ages need to get only 1,000 to 1,333 IU of vitamin A (see RDAs for Vitamin A in ConsumerTips™ for Buying and Using section, page 384). Excess vitamin A in the retinol form is of concern, as it may lead to bone weakening and other problems. *Update:* Hero (February 5, 2007) began providing a letter to inquiring consumers offering to replace the product if from batch number HN60881 manufactured March 2006 (the lot tested by CL) and stating that it was reviewing all aspects of its manufacturing process.

Pet: Pet-Tabs® Complete Daily Vitamin-Mineral Supplement for Dogs contained 1.4 mcg of lead per tablet. *Update:* Virbac (January 19, 2007) issued a news release inaccurately claiming that CL's results were based on a "single test" of their product. In fact, the results were confirmed in a second laboratory prior to publication, per our published protocol. Virbac also claimed to be actively investigating the report, but ten days after this claim, it announced that it had still not completed its investigation. Typically, a lead test can be properly conducted in one day. We would expect Virbac to have announced its findings by now. The release also stated "the level reported is more than 2,800 times below the chronic toxicity level determined safe for dogs..." Virbac's statement suggests that a dog can tolerate approximately 4,000 mcg of lead per day. This is difficult to believe, considering that children may experience lead toxicity at over just 6 mcg per day and adults at less than 100 micrograms per day. CL has not claimed that the amount of lead found in the product is toxic in itself to pets, but recommends that pets, like people, should avoid unnecessary lead exposure.

ConsumerLab.com's testing methods are always immediately available within its reports. CL maintains a cooperative policy to provide manufacturers of failing products detailed test results for their product upon request and the opportunity for re-testing of the tested product by a third party.

Some products, by design, provided specific nutrients at doses above the tolerable upper intake levels (ULs) established by the Institute of Medicine for certain groups of people. Adverse effects—such as skin tingling from niacin, nausea and weakness from magnesium, and immune deficiency and anemia from zinc—may occur when these levels are exceeded for long periods of time. More serious toxicities would not be expected at the doses in these products. Products that exceed the upper limits are footnoted.

See "Testing Methods and Standards," page 657, for more information about the testing and criteria. The test results for 32 supplements (of which ConsumerLab.com selected 23) are listed alphabetically in Test Results for Multivitamin/Multimineral Supplements at the end of this chapter. Nine were tested at the request of their manufacturers/distributors through CL's Voluntary Certification Program and are included for having passed testing. Also listed are seven products similar to ones that passed, but sold under different brand names.

ConsumerTips™ for Buying and Using

In addition to product quality, a critical issue for multivitamin/multimineral products is whether the type of ingredients and amounts are right for the person taking the product. Although by no means comprehensive, below is useful reference information about ingredients often found in multis follows.

As required by the FDA, dietary supplements must show on their labels or packaging the percent of the Daily Value for certain vitamins and minerals contained. However, the percentages given may not reflect the latest Recommended Dietary Allowances (RDAs) or Adequate Intakes (AIs). Nor are products required to provide information indicating whether their ingredients may exceed tolerable upper intake levels (ULs) for the individuals for whom they are intended—many do exceed these ULs.

These values (RDAs, AIs, and ULs) are collectively known as Dietary Reference Intakes (DRIs) and are established by the Institute of Medicine of the National Academies. A Recommended Dietary Allowance (RDA) is the average daily dietary intake level thought to be sufficient to meet the nutrient requirement of nearly all healthy individuals in a particular life stage and gender. An Adequate Intake (AI) is similar to an RDA but is more of an approximation used when there is not sufficient information to develop an RDA. A tolerable upper intake level (UL) is the highest level of daily intake of a nutrient likely to pose no risk of adverse health effects for most people. As intake increases above the UL, the risk of adverse effects may increase. Like the RDAs and AIs, the ULs vary according to one's age, life stage, and gender. Individuals are advised not to regularly exceed the UL unless medically recommended and supervised.

Most products will list the amount of each claimed ingredient. The information provided here can help one determine whether such amounts are appropriate. Keep in mind that 1,000 mcg (micrograms) is the same as 1 mg (milligram), and 1,000 mg equals 1 gram. IU stands for International Units and is used for certain ingredients measured by their activity rather than by weight.

Note that where the text describes what the vitamin does in the body or describes symptoms of severe deficiency, this does not necessarily indicate the benefits to be obtained by taking that vitamin. For example, vitamin A is necessary for vision, but if you are not severely vitamin A deficient, taking more vitamin A will not enhance your vision. Since few people today are severely deficient in *any* nutrient, the actual benefits of nutrient supplementation are more often related to problems caused by marginal deficiency, but these are seldom clear, given the current state of knowledge.

Vitamins and minerals are often used in another way than correcting marginal deficiencies: They are proposed for use at doses much higher than nutritional needs in hopes of providing a benefit that may be unrelated to the nutrient's ordinary function in the body. There are a great many of these proposed megadose uses.

Vitamins

Vitamin A: Vitamin A is necessary to maintain good vision and skin. In supplements, vitamin A usually refers to retinol (including retinyl palmitate and retinyl acetate), as well as beta-carotene. Retinol is found in animal-derived sources, such as dairy foods and liver. Beta-carotene comes from fruits and vegetables, such as carrots and spinach. It is thought that beta-carotene is converted in the body into vitamin A based on the body's need for vitamin A and therefore may be a safer form of vitamin A, by which to avoid potential overdosing. While supplement labels generally combine beta-carotene and retinol in calculating their vitamin A content, many will also note the percent of vitamin A that is contributed by beta-carotene.

Be aware that the amount of vitamin A in supplements is usually shown in IUs. Labels may alternatively (and actually more correctly) list their vitamin A content in micrograms (shown as mcg). The microgram equivalent of one IU of vitamin A depends upon the form of vitamin A. For the retinol form, 0.3 mcg equals 1 IU. For the retinyl acetate form, 3.44 mcg equals 1 IU. For the retinyl palmitate form, .55 micrograms equals 1 IU.

The RDA for vitamin A is 1,000 IU for children 1 to 3 years old, 1,333 IU for those 4 to 8, and 2,000 IU for those 9 to 13. For males 14 years and up, the RDA is 3,000 IU. For females 14 years and older, 2,333 IU is recommended. These amounts can be obtained from the food sources mentioned.

Too much vitamin A can be a problem. The most important risk involves pregnant women: Vitamin A given in modestly excessive doses can cause birth defects. Much higher doses of vitamin A can cause other harm, such as abnormalities in the liver, central nervous system, bone, and skin. The UL for daily intake should not exceed 2,000 IU for children 1 to 3 years old, 3,000 IU for those 4 to 8, 5,666 IU for those under 9 to 13, 9,333 IU for those 14 to 18, and 10,000 IU for adults. To minimize the risk of birth defects such as cleft palate, heart defects, and hydrocephalus, the March of Dimes recommends that a pregnant woman should not use a multivitamin or prenatal supplement that contains more than 5,000 IU of preformed vitamin A. It also advises that a pregnant woman not take any vitamin A supplements beyond that amount and minimize consumption of liver, which contains preformed vitamin A. However, these ULs apply only to vitamin A consumed from supplements, fortified foods, and animal sources, and does not include vitamin A as beta-carotene or intake from fruits and vegetables.

One must be aware that some products, especially those designed for a broad range of individuals, may exceed the ULs for certain subgroups. For example, a multivitamin for children may be appropriate for older children, but exceed ULs for younger children.

B Vitamins: See "B Vitamins," page 317, for more information.

Thiamin (B-1): This B vitamin assists nervous function. It is found in yeast, peas, beans, enriched flour, and whole grains in large enough amounts that supplementation is normally not necessary. The most important exceptions are individuals with alcoholism or congestive heart failure, who may become thiamin deficient. The RDA is 0.5 mg for children 1 to 3, 0.6 mg for those 4 to 8, and 0.9 mg for those 9 to 13. For males 14 years and older, the RDA is 1.2 mg. For females 14 to 18, the RDA is 1.0 mg, and it increases to 1.1 mg for those 19 and older. However, the RDA for pregnant or lactating women is 1.4 mg. ULs have not been established for thiamin, and it is believed to be safe even at very high doses.

Riboflavin (B-2): This B vitamin maintains vision and the skin. Although found in many vegetables and nuts, as well as enriched flour, some supplementation may be needed in children and the elderly. The RDA is 0.5 mg for children 1 to 3, 0.6 mg for those 4 to 8, and 0.9 mg for those 9 to 13. For males 14 years and older, the RDA is 1.3 mg. For females 14 to 18, the RDA is 1.0 mg, and it increases to 1.1 mg for those 19 and older. However, the RDA for pregnant women is 1.4 mg and for lactating women is 1.6 mg. Much higher amounts (400 mg per day) have been suggested in the prevention of migraines. ULs have not been established for riboflavin; this is believed to be a safe nutrient even at high doses.

Niacin (B-3): Niacin helps release energy from carbohydrates. It is available in the diet from enriched white flour, as well as from peanuts, fish, and meat. The RDA is 6 mg for children 1 to 3, 8 mg for those 4 to 8, and 12 mg for those 9 to 13. For males 14 years and older, the RDA is 16 mg. For females 14 and older, the RDA is 14 mg. However, the RDA for pregnant women is 18 mg and for lactating women is 17 mg. High doses of niacin may cause harmless but unpleasant flushing of the skin, including reddening, burning, tingling, itching, and pain. The niacinamide form of niacin is not believed to cause skin flushing. At very high doses of niacin, liver inflammation can also occur. The UL for niacin is fairly low, and is based on the amount causing skin flushing. The UL for niacin applies only to that consumed from supplements and fortified foods (other food sources are not included) and is 10 mg for children 1 to 3, 15 mg for those 4 to 8, 20 mg for those 9 to 13, 30 mg for those 14 to 18, and 35 mg for individuals 19 years and older. Doses of niacin far above the ULs can improve cholesterol levels. Niacin should be used in this way only under medical supervision.

Pyridoxine (B-6): Pyrodoxine is important in many aspects of metabolism, and in maintaining the immune and nervous systems. B-6 is widely available in the diet, but marginal deficiency is believed to be relatively common in the developed world. Inadequate B-6 may raise blood levels of the substance homocysteine, which may increase risk of cardiovascular disease. On this basis, B-6 supplements have been suggested as a means of helping to prevent cardiovascular disease, but efficacy has not been proven. The RDA is 0.5 mg for children 1 to 3, 0.6 mg for those 4 to 8, and 1.0 mg for those 9 to 13.

For males 14 to 50, the RDA is 1.3 mg, and for those 51 and older it is 1.7 mg. For females 14 to 18, it is 1.2 mg, for those 19 to 50, it is 1.3 mg, and for those 51 and older it is 1.5 mg. However, the RDA for pregnant women is 1.9 mg and for lactating women is 2.0 mg. The UL for B-6 is 30 mg for children 1 to 3, 40 mg for those 4 to 8, 60 mg for those 9 to 13, 80 mg for those 14 to 18, and 100 mg for individuals 19 years and older. Intake of B-6 above these levels can cause toxic effects, such as nerve damage. B-6 supplementation at a high but still safe dose of 30 mg daily has shown some promise for treating morning sickness. Other proposed uses of high-dose B-6, such as for PMS, autism, and asthma, lack reliable scientific support.

Folic Acid (Folate, Folacin, or B-9): Folic acid is known to reduce the risk of certain birth defects. Furthermore, adequate folate, along with vitamin B-6 and vitamin B-12, are necessary to keep homocysteine levels low (see B-6). Good natural sources of folic acid include dark green leafy vegetables and oranges. Because folic acid is added to enriched grains and some other foods, most people get sufficient folic acid from their diet. Nonetheless, supplements are generally recommended for women who are pregnant or may soon become pregnant. The RDAs are shown below. It is important to know, however, that these RDAs are based on intake from regular food sources. Folic acid from supplements and fortified foods is actually absorbed twice as well as that from regular food sources. Consequently, if one is relying on supplements or fortified foods to reach the RDA, one needs only half the amount listed in the following RDAs: 150 mcg for children 1 to 3, 200 mcg for children 4 to 8, and 300 mcg for children 9 to 13. For individuals 14 years and older, the RDA is 400 mcg. However, the RDA for pregnant women is 600 mcg, and for lactating women is 500 mcg. In view of folic acid's importance to developing fetuses during the first few weeks after conception, it is recommended that all women capable of becoming pregnant consume 400 mcg from supplements or fortified foods in addition to intake of food folic acid from a varied diet.

The UL for folic acid applies only to that consumed from supplements and fortified foods and is 300 mcg for children 1 to 3, 400 mcg for those 4 to 8, 600 mcg for those 9 to 13, and 800 mcg for those 14 to 18. For individuals 19 years and older, the UL is 1,000 mcg. Intake of high doses of folic acid can make it difficult to detect severe vitamin B-12 deficiency, which is a relatively rare condition; however, missing the diagnosis can be catastrophic, and that possibility is the main reason for concern about excessive folic acid intake.

B-12: Vitamin B-12 deficiency can cause anemia, and if the deficiency is severe enough, irreversible nerve damage may occur. B-12 is also required, along with folate and B-6, to maintain low homocysteine levels. However, true deficiency of this vitamin is rare. Vitamin B-12 is found in abundant quantity in meat, dairy products, and eggs, and the body can store enough B-12 to last for years. Note, though, that B-12 is not found at useful levels in any purely plant-based substance. For this reason, total vegetarians (*vegans*) need to take a B-12 supplement. Deficiency may also occur in people with low stomach acidity, such as seniors or those taking drugs that reduce stomach acid, such as Prilosec or Zantac. The reason is that stomach acid is required to separate B-12 from the proteins in which it is naturally found. People with low stomach acid can still absorb the purified B-12 found in supplements. The RDA is 0.9 mcg for children 1 to 3, 1.2 mcg for those 4 to 8, and 1.8 mcg for those 9 to 13. For individuals 14 years and older, the RDA is 2.4 mcg. However, the RDA for pregnant women is 2.6 mcg and for lactating women is 2.8 mcg. ULs have not been established for vitamin B-12.

Vitamin C (ascorbic acid): See also "Vitamin C," page 412.
Vitamin C is required for healthy blood vessel walls, gums, and bones. It is also a strong antioxidant. Vitamin C is found in many vegetables, such as broccoli and Brussels sprouts, as well citrus and other fruits; a healthful diet should allow one to meet the RDA. The RDA is 15 mg for children 1 to 3, 25 mg for those 4 to 8, and 45 mg for those 9 to 13. For males 14 to 18, the RDA is 75 mg, and it is 90 mg for those ages 19 and higher. For females 14 to 18, the RDA is 65 mg, and it is 75 mg for those ages 19 and higher. However, the RDA for pregnant women 18 years and younger is 80 mg, and 85 mg if 19 or older, and the RDA for lactating women 18 years and younger is 115 mg, and 120 mg if 19 or older. Too much vitamin C can cause diarrhea and other gastric disturbances. The UL for vitamin C is 400 mg for children 1 to 3, 650 mg for those 4 to 8, 1,200 mg for those 9 to 13, 1,800 mg for those 14 to 18, and 2,000 mg for individuals 19 years and older. Dosages of vitamin C far above nutritional needs have been recommended for a great many illnesses, including the common cold.

Vitamin D (cholecalciferol): See also "Bone-Health Supplements: Calcium and Vitamin D," page 31, volume 1.

Vitamin D helps the body absorb calcium to promote strong bones and teeth. It can be obtained in sufficient amounts from fortified milks and foods and from exposure to sunlight. However, people who live in northern climates may easily become vitamin D deficient during the winter, especially if they are dark-skinned. Also, increased concern about skin cancer has caused people to avoid the sun, which creates a potential risk of reduced vitamin D. There is some evidence that inadequate vitamin D intake can lead to an increased risk of various forms of cancer, including breast cancer. Vitamin D is measured as micrograms of cholecalciferol or in International Units (IUs) of vitamin D activity. One microgram equals 40 IUs. An AI (Adequate Intake) has been established, but is relevant only if an individual is not getting adequate exposure to sunlight. The AI is 5 micrograms (200 IU) for individuals ages 1 to 50, 10 micrograms (400 IU) for those 51 to 70, and 15 micrograms (600 IU) for those 71 years and older. Excessive intake of vitamin D as a supplement may result in hypercalcemia (too much calcium in the blood) with symptoms including constipation, confusion, weakness, loss of appetite, and painful calcium deposit. Taking too much during pregnancy can cause abnormalities in the fetus. The UL for individuals 1 year old and above is 50 micrograms (2,000 IU).

Vitamin E (tocopherol): See also "Vitamin E Supplements and Skin Care Products," page 422.

Vitamin E is an antioxidant. Most diets provide enough vitamin E to meet RDAs, as it is easily obtained from food sources such as nuts, seeds, whole grains, vegetable oils, and fatty meat. For a time, megadoses of this nutrient (much higher than could be reasonably obtained through diet) were widely recommended in the belief that it would help prevent cancer and cardiovascular disease. Unfortunately, accumulating evidence has largely dashed this hope, at least regarding the most common form of vitamin E supplements (alpha-tocopherol, whether synthetic or natural). There is still some possibility that high dosages of vitamin E may reduce risk of prostate cancer, and that other forms of vitamin E, such as gamma-tocopherol, might offer the benefits hoped for with standard vitamin E supplements. High-dose vitamin E has also shown promise for slowing the progress of Alzheimer's disease and enhancing the immune response to vaccinations in seniors. There are literally hundreds of other proposed uses of high-dose vitamin E, but they generally lack strong scientific support. Vitamin E is measured as IUs of vitamin E activity or, more recently, in milligrams of active alpha-tocopherol. Most supplements are still labeled using IUs. Complicating matters a bit, the conversion factor between IUs and milligrams differs for natural vitamin E versus synthetic vitamin E. Most multis contain synthetic vitamin E, for which the conversion rate is 1 IU for each 0.45 mg of active alpha-tocopherol. The conversion rate for natural vitamin E is 1 IU for each 0.67 mg of active alpha-tocopherol.

The RDA for vitamin E as active alpha-tocopherol for children 1 to 3 is 6 mg (13 IU synthetic or 9 IU natural), for those 4 to 8 it is 7 mg (16 IU synthetic or 10 IU natural), and for those 9 to 13 it is 11 mg (24 IU synthetic or 16 IU natural). The RDA for individuals ages 14 and older is 15 mg (33 IU synthetic or 22 IU natural). However, the RDA for lactating women is 19 mg (42 IU synthetic or 28 IU natural). There are some concerns that high doses of vitamin E may impair platelet activity and lead to increased risk of bleeding. This risk would be expected to increase if high doses of vitamin E were combined with drugs that impair clotting. The ULs for vitamin E apply only to that consumed from supplements and fortified foods and are as follows: for children 1 to 3, it is 200 mg, for children 4 to 8, it is 300 mg, for those 9 to 13 it is 600 mg, and for those 14 to 18, it is 800 mg. The UL for individuals 19 and older is 1,000 mg. One must also be aware that the 1,000 mg per day adult UL translates into about 1,500 IUs of natural vitamin E, but only 1,100 IUs of synthetic vitamin E because both the active and the inactive forms of alpha-tocopherol found in synthetic vitamin E may contribute to this effect on blood clotting. The ULs therefore translate approximately into the following IU amounts: for children 1 to 3, the UL is 220 IU synthetic or 300 IU natural, for those 4 to 8, it is 330 IU synthetic or 450 IU natural, for those 9 to 13, it is 660 IU synthetic or 900 IU natural, and for those 14 to 18, it is 880 IU synthetic or 1,200 IU natural. (See "Vitamin E Supplements and Skin Care Products," page 422).

Vitamin K: Vitamin K plays a central role in blood clotting as well as bone formation. Foods like green leafy vegetables can provide sufficient amounts, and intestinal bacteria also produce vitamin K. True deficiency is rare; however, there is some evidence that vitamin K supplements at doses higher than nutritional needs may help fight osteoporosis. The AI (Adequate Intake) of vitamin K is measured in micrograms (shown as mcg). The AI is 30 mcg for children ages 1 to 3, 55 mcg for children 4 to 8, 60 mcg for those ages 9 to 13, and 75 mcg for those ages 14 to 18. For males 19 years and older, it is 120 mcg. For females 19 years and older, it is 90 mcg. There is no UL established for vitamin K.

Minerals and Other Ingredients:

Calcium: See also "Bone-Health Supplements: Calcium and Vitamin D," page 31, volume 1.

While critical for strong bones and teeth, calcium is a very bulky material, and most multis therefore do not contain the total recommended daily intake amount in a tablet, as it might make the tablet too large. Consequently, one should consider getting calcium from a separate calcium supplement or fortified food or beverage. The AI for calcium is 500 mg for children 1 to 3, 800 mg for children 4 to 8, and 1,300 mg for children 9 to 18. For adults aged 19 to 50, it is 1,000 mg. For those 51 years and older, it is 1,200 mg per day. The UL for calcium is 2,500 mg and applies to all individuals 1 year and older. Excessive use of calcium supplements might raise risk of kidney and bladder stones.

Chromium: See also "Chromium," page 352.

Chromium plays a role in the body's regulation of blood sugar. Chromium is found in liver and whole-wheat products. It is unclear whether marginal chromium deficiency occurs commonly or rarely. Chromium supplementation (especially in doses considerably above nutritional needs) has shown some promise for helping to regulate blood-sugar levels in people with type 2 diabetes. Chromium is also sold as a weight-loss aid, but there is little evidence that it really works. AIs for chromium are measured in micrograms (shown as mcg) and are: 11 mcg for children ages 1 to 3, and 15 mcg for children ages 4 to 8. For boys ages 9 to 13, it is 25 mcg, while for girls it is 21 mcg. For males ages 14 to 50, it is 35 mcg. For females ages 14 to 18, it is 24 mcg, rising to 25 mcg for those ages 19 to 50. For men 51 years and older, it is 30 mcg, and for women aged 51 and older, it is 20 mcg. Women who are pregnant need more: 29 mcg if 18 or younger and 30 mcg if 19 and older. Lactating women need even more: 44 mcg if 18 or younger and 45 mcg if 19 or older. There is no UL established for chromium, but there are concerns that excessive intake could cause kidney and other organ damage in certain people.

Copper: Copper is necessary for proper development of connective tissue, nerve coverings, and skin pigment. Copper is found in foods such as organ meats, oysters, nuts, and seeds and can be obtained in sufficient quantity from a good diet. People who take zinc supplements may need to take extra copper. Copper in supplements may be shown in milligrams (mg) or micrograms (shown as mcg). One milligram is equal to 1,000 micrograms. The RDAs are:

340 mcg for children ages 1 to 3, 440 mcg for children ages 4 to 8, 700 mcg for those ages 9 to 13, 890 mcg for those 14 to 18. For people over 19 years of age, the RDA is 900 mcg. For women who are pregnant the RDA is 1,000 mcg, while for lactating women it is 1,300 mcg. Excessive consumption of copper may cause nausea and liver damage. The daily upper limits for copper are 1,000 mcg for children ages 1 to 3, 3,000 mcg for those 4 to 8, 5,000 mcg for those 9 to 13, 8,000 mcg for those 14 to 18, and 10,000 mcg for people 19 years and older. It is also worth noting that a recent study found an association between excess copper intake and accelerated mental decline: People over age 65 who consumed and average 2,750 mcg of copper per day and had diets high in saturated and trans fats suffered mental decline almost 1.5 times as great as people with similar diets, but who averaged only 880 mg of copper per day. Another good reason to limit copper intake.

Animal studies have shown that one form of copper called copper (or *cupric*) oxide may not be well absorbed. Other forms, such as copper sulfate, cupric acetate, and alkaline copper carbonate, may, therefore, be preferable. Unfortunately, copper oxide is common in supplements (including some that have passed CL's testing) because it is less bulky and allows for smaller pills.

Iodine: Iodine is needed for making thyroid hormones, and iodine deficiency causes *hypothyroidism* (low thyroid). However, iodine deficiency is uncommon in the developed world, and too much iodine can also cause hypothyroidism! Seafood and seaweeds provide iodine. In addition, most table salt is now iodized and represents a good dietary source of iodine. The RDAs are given in micrograms (shown as mcg) and are: 90 mcg for children ages 1 to 8, and 120 mcg for children ages 9 to 13. For both males and females ages 14 and older, the RDA is 150 mcg. However, for pregnant women it is 220 mcg, and for lactating women it is 290 mcg. Too much iodine taken during pregnancy can cause problems in infants. ULs for iodine are: 200 mcg for children ages 1 to 3, 300 mcg for those 4 to 8, 600 mcg for those 9 to 13, 900 mcg for those 14 to 18, and 1,100 mcg for all 19 years and older.

Iron: See also "Iron," page 360. Iron deficiency is the leading cause of anemia. Deficiency is most common in menstruating woman, and is also seen in some children and pregnant women. Adult men are seldom deficient in iron, and many multivitamins for adult men specifically leave out iron because there are concerns that excess iron intake might increase risk of heart disease. Meat, poultry, and fish are rich in iron. Dried fruits, grains, and green leafy vegetables are also good sources, although iron from plant sources is absorbed only half as well as that from animal sources. The RDA is 7 mg for children 1 to 3 years, and 10 mg for those 4 to 8. It then falls to 8 mg for those 9 to 13. For males 14 to 18, it is 11 mg, and for those 19 years and older, the RDA again falls to 8 mg. For females 14 to 18, it is 15 mg, and for those 19 to 50, it is 18 mg, falling to 8 mg for women ages 51 and higher. However, because of the needs of the fetus, the RDA for pregnant women is increased to 27 mg. For lactating women 18 years old and younger, the RDA is 10 mg, and 9 mg for lactating women 19 and older. Also, postmenopausal women taking hormone replacement therapy may need more iron if the therapy causes periodic uterine bleeding. Oral contraceptives may reduce menstrual blood losses, so women taking them may need less daily iron. High daily amounts of iron can cause gastrointestinal distress, especially when consuming iron supplements on an empty stomach. The UL is 40 mg for children 13 years and younger, and 45 mg for all others. However, these limits may be too high for people with hereditary hemochomatosis, who are at risk for accumulating harmful levels of iron.

Magnesium: See also "Magnesium," page 370.

Magnesium assists metabolism and the nervous system. There is some controversy regarding whether marginal magnesium deficiency is a rare or a common occurrence. Whole grains, nuts, and beans are good sources of magnesium. The RDA is 80 mg for children 1 to 3, 130 mg for those 4 to 8, and 240 mg for those 9 to 13. For males 14 to 18, it is 410 mg, for those 19 to 30, it falls to 400 mg, and for those 31 years and older, it is 420 mg. For females 14 to 18, it is 360 mg, for those 19 to 30, it falls to 310 mg, and for those 31 years and older, it is 320 mg. However, for pregnant women it is 400 mg if 18 years or younger, 350 mg if 19 to 30, and 360 mg if 31 or older. For lactating women, it is 360 mg if 18 years or younger, 310 mg if 19 to 30, and 320 mg if 31 or older. People with diabetes are thought to have an increased need for magnesium. Magnesium supplements around or above the levels of the ULs have shown some promise for the treatment of migraine headaches and high blood pressure, as well for preventing kidney stones. Excessive magnesium intake can cause nausea and vomiting, low blood pressure, and muscle weakness. The UL for magnesium applies only to that consumed from supplements or other medication and is 65 mg for children 1 to 3 and 110 mg for those 4 to 8. For individuals 9 years and older, the UL is 350 mg.

Manganese: Manganese is involved in bone formation and metabolism. Nuts, legumes, tea, and whole grains are rich sources of manganese and can provide adequate amounts. The daily AI for manganese is 1.2 mg for children 1 to 3 years, and 1.5 mg for those 4 to 8. It is 1.9 mg for males 9 to 13, 2.2 mg for those 14 to 18, and 2.3 mg for those 19 years and older. For females 9 to 18, the level is 1.6 mg, increasing to 1.8 mg for those 19 years and older. Pregnant women need 2.0 mg per day and lactating women need 2.6 mg per day. Too much manganese may cause neurological side effects. The UL for manganese is 2 mg for children 1 to 3, 3 mg for children 4 to 8, 6 mg for children 9 to 13, and 9 mg for children 14 to 18. The UL for adults 19 years and older is 11 mg.

Molybdenum: Molybdenum is a constituent of various enzymes in the body, and can be obtained from legumes, grain products, and nuts. Deficiency is rare in the U.S. RDAs for molybdenum are given in micrograms (shown as mcg) and are: 17 mcg for children 1 to 3 years, 22 mcg for those 4 to 8, 34 mcg for those 9 to 13, and 43 mcg for those 14 to 18. Individuals 19 years and older need 45 mcg per day; women who are pregnant or nursing should get 50 mcg per day. Massive amounts of molybdenum can cause goutlike symptoms. The UL for molybdenum is 300 mcg for children 1 to 3, 600 mcg for those 4 to 8, 1,100 mcg for those 9 to 13, 1,700 mcg for those 14 to 18, and 2,000 mcg for those 19 years and older.

Selenium: See also "Cancer-Prevention Supplements: Green Tea, Lycopene, and Selenium," see page 45, volume 1.

Selenium is used by the body in it its antioxidant system. There is some preliminary evidence that selenium supplements may help prevent certain forms of cancer, but this benefit appears to be limited to those who are deficient in the mineral, and deficiency is thought to be relatively uncommon in the developed world. Foods containing selenium include nuts, wheat germ, whole wheat, and orange juice. The RDA is 20 mcg for children 1 to 3, 30 mcg for those 4 to 8, and 40 mcg for those 9 to 13. For individuals 14 and older, the RDA is 55 mcg. However, the RDA for pregnant women is 60 mcg and, for nursing women, is 70 mcg per day. At very high doses, selenium can cause hair loss and tissue damage. The UL for selenium is 90 mcg for children 1 to 3, 150 mcg for those 4 to 8, and 280 mcg for those 9 to 13. The UL for individuals 19 years and older is 400 mcg.

Zinc: See also "Zinc Supplements (Lozenges, Pills, and Liquids)," page 439.

Zinc plays a role in brain function, wound healing, and sperm production. Many breakfast cereals are fortified with zinc, which is naturally abundant in red meats, certain seafood, and whole grains. However, mild zinc deficiency is thought to be fairly common. Zinc supplements at nutritional doses may enhance immunity in people who are significantly deficient in the mineral, such as seniors in nursing homes and people who live in developing countries. The RDA of zinc is 3 mg for children ages 1 to 3, 5 mg for those 4 to 8, and 8 mg for those 9 to 13. For males 14 and older, the RDA is 11 mg. For females 14 to 18, it is 9 mg, while for those 19 years and older, it is 8 mg per day. The RDA for pregnant women who are 18 years or younger is 13 mg, while it is 11 mg for pregnant women 19 years and older. For lactating women, the RDAs are 14 mg if 18 years and younger, or 12 mg if 19 years or older. High doses of zinc have shown promise for treatment of acne, macular degeneration, and sickle cell disease. However, too much zinc can be toxic, and people have caused harm to themselves using zinc for these conditions. Excessive zinc impairs the absorption of copper and can cause immune deficiency, heart problems, and anemia. Weak evidence associates long-term zinc supplementation at high doses (over 100 mg per day) with an increased risk of prostate cancer.

ULs for zinc are: 7 mg for children ages 1 to 3, 12 mg for those 4 to 8, 23 mg for those 9 to 13, 34 mg for those 14 to 18, and 40 mg for individuals 19 years and older. NOTE: Zinc is widely used in an entirely different manner for treatment of colds: in the form of a lozenge or nasal spray to kill viruses. This use has no relationship to the effects of zinc taken as an oral supplement.

Test Results for Multivitamin/Multimineral Supplements

Product and Dose‡ Manufacturer (Mf) or Distributor (Dist) Test Results	Test Results			
	Approved or not approved	Contained claimed amount of nutrients	Acceptable level for lead	Broke apart properly
General (Adult)				
Eniva® VIBE™ (1 oz packet per day) Dist: Eniva Corp.	*not* approved	Only 54.2% of claimed 5000 IU of vitamin A	✔	N/A
Floradix® Epresat® Multivitamin, Liquid Extract Formula (10 mL per day) Mf: Salus-Haus	approved	✔	✔	N/A
The Greatest Vitamin in the World (9 capsules per day) Dist: The Greatest Vitamin in the World	*not* approved**[1] (Above UL for magnesium)	Only 85% of claimed 800 mcg of folate per capsule	✔	N/A
Healthy Moments™ Mint Cream Flavor Vitamin Strips Multi-Vitamin (2 strips per day) Dist: Momentus Solutions, LLC	*not* approved	No Vitamin A found—claimed 75 mcg (137 IU per strip); 180% of claimed 2 mg of niacin per strip	✔	N/A
Kirkland Signature™ Daily Multi, With Lycopene & Lutein and Calcium (1 tablet per day) Dist: Costco Wholesale Corporation	approved	✔	✔	✔

continued

Product and Dose	Test Results			
	Approval	**Contained claimed**	**Acceptable level**	**Broke apart**
Nutrilite® Daily (1 tablet per day)* Dist: Access Business Group International LLC	approved	✔	✔	✔
Nutrilite® Double X™ Multivitamin, Multimineral, Phytonutrient (2 of each, a gold, silver and bronze tablet per day)* Dist: Access Business Group International LLC	approved**[1] (Above UL for niacin)	✔	✔	✔
Pharmanex® LifePak® Dietary Supplement, New! Anti-Aging Formula (2 packets per day)* Dist: Pharmanex, LLC	approved Also approved for alpha-lipoic acid, B vitamins, vitamin C, and vita-min E	✔	✔	N/A
Swanson® Daily Multi-Vitamin & Mineral (1–2 capsules per day) Dist: Swanson Health Products	*not* approved**[1] (Above ULs for niacin at 1 capsule and vitamin A at 2 capsules)	Only 77.5% of claimed 400 mcg of folate per capsule	✔	N/A
Vitamin World® One Take-One®, Time Release (1 tablet per day)* Mf: Vitamin World, Inc.	approved**[1] (Above UL for niacin)	✔	✔	N/A

Product and Dose	Test Results			
	Approval	Contained claimed	Acceptable level	Broke apart
Vitamin World® Time Release Mega Vita-Min™ Long Acting Formula (1 tablet per day)* Mf: Vitamin World, Inc.	approved**[1] (Above UL for niacin)	✔	✔	N/A
Weil™ Andrew Weil, M.D. Daily Multivitamin for Optimum Health (1 tablet per day) Dist: Weil Nutritional Supplements	**not** approved**[1] (Above UL for niacin)	Only 73% of claimed 10,000 IU of vitamin A (as beta-carotene); 251% of claimed 60 mg of calcium	✔	✔

Similar to Approved Products***

Puritan's Pride Time Release Complete One®, Long Acting

Mf: Puritan's Pride, Inc.

Puritan's Pride Time Release Mega Vita-Min™, Long Acting Formula

Mf: Puritan's Pride, Inc.

Prenatal

Product and Dose	Approval	Contained claimed	Acceptable level	Broke apart
Pregnancy Plus™ Multivitamin Formulated by Fertility Specialist Amos Grunebaum, MD (1 tablet per day) Dist: Fairhaven Health, LLC	approved	✔	✔	✔
TwinLab® Pre-natal Care Multi Vitamin Caps (2 capsules per day) Mfd by Ideasphere, Inc.	approved**[1] (Above UL for niacin)	✔	✔	✔

continued

Product and Dose	Test Results			
	Approval	Contained claimed	Acceptable level	Broke apart
Women's				
Nature's Plus® The Energy Supplements® Especially Yours® Women's Multi-Vitamin Supplement (3 tablets per day) Mf: Natural Organics Laboratories, Inc.	*not* approved	292% of claimed 50 mg of calcium per tablet	✔	Failed to break apart properly
One A Day® Women's Multivitamin/Multimineral Supplement (1 tablet per day) Dist: Bayer HealthCare, LLC	approved	✔	✔	✔
The Vitamin Shoppe® Multivitamins Especially for Women (2 tablets per day) Dist: The Vitamin Shoppe	*not* approved	Only 54% of claimed 100 mg of calcium per tablet	Lead con-tamination at 15.3 mcg/day	✔
Vitamin World® Time Release Mega Vita Min For Women (2 tablets per day)* Mf: Vitamin World, Inc.	approved** (Above UL for niacin)	✔	✔	N/A
Similar to Approved Products* **				

Puritan's Pride® Time Release Mega Vita Min for Women

Mf: Puritan's Pride, Inc.

Product and Dose	Test Results			
	Approval	Contained claimed	Acceptable level	Broke apart
Men				
NOW® Adam™ Superior Men's Multi with Saw Palmetto, Lycopene, Lutein, CoQ10, ZMA®, & Ginkgo Biloba (2 tablets per day) Mf: NOW Foods	*not* approved**[1] (Above UL for niacin)	✔	✔	Failed to break apart properly
Vitamin World® High Potency Time Release Ultra Vita Man™ (2 tablets per day)* Mf: Vitamin World, Inc.	approved	✔	✔	N/A
Win™ Fuel Men's Formula (1 tablet per day) Dist: WinFuel, Inc.	*not* approved	Only 81% of claimed 4,000 IU of vitamin A; only 75% of claimed 400 mcg of folate	✔	✔
Similar to Approved Products*				
Nature's Bounty® High Potency Time Release, Ultra Man™ Mf: Nature's Bounty, Inc.				
Puritan's Pride® High Potency Time Release Ultra Vita Man™ Mf: Puritan's Pride, Inc.				
Seniors				
AARP Maturity Formula® (1 tablet per day) Dist: United Healthcare Products, LLC	*not* approved	✔	✔	Failed to break apart properly

continued

Product and Dose	Test Results			
	Approval	**Contained claimed**	**Acceptable level**	**Broke apart**
Centrum® Silver® Specially Formulated Multivitamin/ Multimineral Supplement for Adults 50+, Now with Lycopene, Improved Formula (1 tablet per day) Dist: Wyeth Consumer Healthcare	approved	✔	✔	✔
Member's Mark® Complete Multi, Now With Lycopene, USP (1 tablet per day) Dist: Sam's West, Inc.	approved	✔	✔	✔
One Source Complete® 50 Plus Advanced Multivitamin and Mineral for Adults 50+, Improved Formula (1 caplet per day) Mf: Perrigo Co.	approved	✔	✔	✔
Puritan's Pride® ABC Plus® Senior, Multi-Vitamin Multi-Mineral Formula, with Lutein and Lycopene, Iron Free Formula (1 tablet per day)* Mf: Puritan's Pride, Inc.	approved	✔	✔	N/A

Similar to Approved Products*

Vitamin World® ABC Plus® Senior, Multi-Vitamin Multi-Mineral Formula, with Lutein and Lycopene, Iron Free Formula

Dist: Vitamin World, Inc.

Multivitamin/Multimineral Supplements

Product and Dose	Test Results			
	Approval	Contained claimed	Acceptable level	Broke apart
Children's				
Dr. Fuhrman™ Pixie-Vites™ Children's Multi-Vitamin Wild Berry Blast (under 12 yrs, 1 stick per day; over 12 yrs 2 sticks per day) Dist: Dr. Fuhrman online	approved**[1] Above UL for magnesium (ages 1 to 3)	✔	✔	N/A
Flintstones™ Complete, Children's Multivitamin/ Multimineral Supplement (2–3 yrs—½ chewable tablet per day; over 4 yrs—1 tablet per day) Dist: Bayer HealthCare LLC	approved	✔	✔	N/A
Hero Nutritionals™ Yummi® Bears® Multi-Vitamin and Mineral (up to 3 bears per day) Dist: Hero Nutritional Products, LLC	***not* approved** At 3 bears per day, above UL for vitamin A (ages 1 to 8) and zinc (ages 1 to 3)	216% of claimed IU of vitamin A per bear; 211% of claimed 3 mg of calcium per bear	✔	N/A
Puritan's Pride Children's Multi Gummies (2 gummies per day)* Dist: Puritan's Pride, Inc	approved	✔	✔	N/A

continued

403

Product and Dose	Test Results			
	Approval	Contained claimed	Acceptable level	Broke apart
Similar to Approved Products***				
Vitamin World® Children's Multi Gummies Dist: Vitamin World, Inc				
Pet				
21st Century Pet Nutrition Pet Chews™ Plus (1 chewable tablet per day if 10 lbs and over; ½ tablet if under 10 lbs) Dist: 21st Century Pet Nutrition	approved	✔	✔	N/A
Pet-Tabs® Complete Daily Vitamin-Mineral Supplement for Dogs (1 chewable tablet per day if 10 lbs and over; ½ tablet if under 10 lbs) Dist: Virback AH, Inc.	***not* approved**	✔	Contained lead (1.41 mcg per tablet)	N/A

‡ See also "More Brand Information," page 675.

*Tested through CL's Voluntary Certification Program prior to, at time of, or after initial posting of this Product Review.

N/A—Not applicable.

**Exceeds the UL for one or more nutrients.

***Product identical in formulation and manufacture to a product that has passed testing but sold under a different brand. For more information on CL's Multi-Label Testing Program see "Selection and Testing," page 25, volume 1.

✔ Check indicates the results met the criteria listed in the column heading.

[1] According to the label, all or most of the niacin in this product is in the niacinamide form. Although the product exceeds the UL for niacin, the UL is based on niacin's potential for skin flushing and tingling—side effects not associated with this form of niacin. Other side effects associated with niacin may, however, occur at doses much higher than those suggested on the label.

Potassium

Potassium is an essential mineral that is found in foods and supplements in many forms, including potassium bicarbonate, potassium citrate, potassium gluconate, potassium acetate, and (particularly in salt substitutes) potassium chloride. Similarly, potassium is often used in supplements to stabilize other elements, such as in potassium iodide supplements, where potassium stabilizes iodine as a radioprotective agent. (See ConsumerTips™ for Buying and Using, page 406, and "Nuclear Radiation Protection Supplements: Potassium Iodide [KI] and Potassium Iodate [KIO_3]," page 152, volume 1.)

Potassium, like sodium and chloride, is an important electrolyte in your body; it's involved in the proper functioning of your nervous system, skeletal system, cardiac muscle, and metabolism. It also helps maintain normal blood pressure.

Most people get enough potassium from their diets, so potassium supplements are typically used only to treat or prevent a potassium deficiency caused from excessive potassium loss. Causes of potassium deficiency include the use of diuretic drugs ("water pills") to treat high blood pressure, prolonged vomiting, diarrhea, or laxative abuse. Deficiency can cause muscle weakness, irregular heartbeat, listlessness, mood changes, irrational behavior, nausea, and vomiting. Potassium may help reduce hypertension, particularly in people who consume too much sodium.

Quality Concerns and Product Testing

Like other supplements, neither the FDA nor any other federal or state agency routinely tests potassium products for quality prior to sale. However, quality issues for potassium supplements can include the following:

Labeled Amount: Does the product really contain the labeled amount of potassium? Too little potassium in a supplement is a problem if you're relying on it to prevent or correct a deficiency. Avoid excessive consumption of potassium if you have kidney disease.

Purity: Like other minerals, many sources of potassium may naturally contain amounts of heavy metals such as lead. In fetuses, infants, and children even low levels of lead can adversely affect neurobehavioral development and cognitive function. In adults, lead at somewhat higher levels can cause elevated blood pressure and anemia, and adversely affect the nervous and reproductive systems. Lead is of particular concern during pregnancy as the mother can transfer it to her fetus. Previous testing of potassium supplements by ConsumerLab.com found one product with excessive lead. Even a small amount of lead contamination can become a problem because of the large doses of potassium taken to treat deficiencies.

Availability: Once in your body, will the pill break down, or disintegrate properly so that it can release its contents?

ConsumerLab.com, as part of its mission to independently evaluate products that affect health, wellness, and nutrition, purchased many leading potassium supplements products sold in the U.S. and tested them to determine whether they 1) possessed the claimed amount of potassium, 2) could disintegrate properly in order to release their contents for absorption, and 3) were free of unacceptable levels of lead (see the appropriate section in "ConsumerLab.com's Testing Methods and Standards," page 659).

Test Findings

All of the products contained their claimed amounts of potassium and all tablets and caplets disintegrated properly when tested. In addition, none of the products exceeded acceptable levels of lead.

Products varied in the type of potassium used, and the prices ranged from about 3 cents to more than 20 cents for the same amount of potassium (99 mg).

The 13 products that were selected for testing and a summary of the results are listed alphabetically in Test Results for Potassium Supplements. Also included in the list are 3 other products (indicated with an asterisk) that have met the same criteria through CL's Voluntary Certification Program (see Selection and Testing, page 25, volume 1).

ConsumerTips™ for Buying and Using

To determine the amount of potassium in a product, read the Supplement Facts panel carefully. A product, for example, named "Potassium Gluconate 550 mg" will actually contain only about 90 mg of actual, or elemental, potassium because potassium makes up less than half of the weight of most potassium compounds. For instance, potassium makes up only 16.7% of the weight of potassium gluconate, 38.3% in potassium citrate, and 52% in potassium chloride.

When sold as dietary supplements, potassium pills may contain up to 99 mg of elemental potassium/pill. Products containing as much as 800 mg of potassium/tablet, however, are available by prescription only, as is potassium in the form of liquid, powder, granules, or dissolving tablets for preparation in a solution or suspension. Such products may be preferable when high doses are needed. (Sometimes you see potassium dosages calculated in milliequivalents [1 milliequivalent equals 39.09 milligrams of potassium].)

More than 90% of potassium is absorbed in the gastrointestinal tract and nearly all of the common forms of potassium are absorbed equally well. Some minor differences among the forms are as follows: Potassium chloride, unless properly processed, is most likely to have the greatest amounts of lead; potassium citrate may be most helpful for reducing blood pressure; and potassium gluconate has the least bitter taste.

Because lack of dietary potassium is rare, there is no recommended daily allowance (RDA) for potassium, although adults should get a minimum of 1,600 mg to 2,000 mg of potassium a day and children should get at least 1,000 mg a day. Foods especially rich in potassium (containing more than 300 milligrams of potassium a serving) are acorn or butternut squash, potatoes (with skin), spinach, bananas, orange juice, avocados, lima beans, cantaloupes, peaches, tomatoes, flounder, salmon, and cod. Some salt substitutes also contain high amounts of potassium. (An extensive listing of potassium levels in foods is available from the USDA as a PDF document at http://www.nal.usda.gov/fnic/foodcomp/Data/SR17/wtrank/sr17a306.pdf.)

For treating potassium deficiency or preventing potassium loss, the daily potassium dose for adults is 200 to 400 mg (5 to 10 milliequivalents) taken three to four times a day, for a total daily dose ranging from 600 mg to 1,600 mg. A physician should determine children's doses. Because supplements cannot contain more than 99 mg of potassium/tablet, you would have to take many pills to reach the prescribed dose. You should consider, therefore, using a prescription product, which provides more potassium per dosage unit.

Potassium from supplements can cause diarrhea, nausea, stomach pain, mild gas, and vomiting, although these side effects may be reduced when potassium is taken with meals. More serious side effects, though less common, include confusion, irregular heartbeat, numbness or tingling in hands, feet, or lips, shortness of breath, anxiety, tiredness or weakness. Supplements can also cause more severe stomach pain, chest or throat pain when swallowing.

Tolerable Upper Intake Levels (UL) has not been established for potassium because your body excretes excess potassium as long as your kidneys are healthy.

When taking potassium supplements, you should increase your intake of magnesium (see "Magnesium," page 370). Many potassium products contain magnesium stearate, which improves the consistency of the product during manufacturing, but it is not a significant source of magnesium.

Concerns and Cautions

Individuals with kidney disease cannot properly control levels of electrolytes in their body; for this reason, the use of potassium (or any other mineral) can be dangerous and should be used only under medical supervision.

Individuals taking potassium-sparing diuretics (such as spironolactone), ACE inhibitors (such as captopril), or trimethoprim/sulfamethoxazole should not take potassium supplements without medical supervision; dangerous levels of potassium may develop when the drugs and diuretics interact. Liberal use of salt substitutes that contain potassium chloride can cause a potassium overload in people with kidney disease.

Test Results for Potassium Supplements

Product (label info: form and amount of elemental potassium, dosing)‡ Manufacturer (Mf) or distributor (Dist)	Test Results		
	Approved or not approved	Contained labeled amount of potassium	Acceptable level of lead
Carlson® Complexed Potassium (potassium glycinate complex 99 mg/ tablet, 1/day) Dist: Carlson Division of J.R. Carlson Laboratories, Inc.	approved	✔	✔
Doctor's Trust™ Vitamins, Potassium, 99 mg (potassium gluconate 99 mg/tablet, 2/day) Doctor's Trust Vitamins	approved	✔	✔
Equaline™ natural potassium gluconate 550 mg (potassium gluconate 90 mg/tablet, 1/day) Dist: Albertsons	approved	✔	✔
Natural Factors® Potassium Citrate 99 mg (potassium citrate 99 mg/tablet, 1–5/day) Mf: Natural Factors, Canada	approved	✔	✔
NutriCology® Potassium Citrate, Hypoallergenic (potassium citrate 99 mg/ capsule, 1/day) Dist: NutriCology, Inc.	approved	✔	✔

continued

Product (label info.)	Test Results		
	Approval	Contained labeled	Acceptable level
Pure Encapsulations® Potassium (aspartate) (potassium aspartate 99 mg/ capsule, 2/day) Mf: pure encapsulations, inc.	approved	✔	✔
Puritan's Pride® Potassium Magnesium Aspartate* (potassium aspartate 50 mg/ tablet, 1/day) Mf: Puritan's Pride, Inc.	approved	✔	✔
Rite Aid Potassium Gluconate (potassium gluconate 99 mg/ tablet, 1/day) Dist: Rite Aid Corporation	approved	✔	✔
Sundown® Benefits Potassium Gluconate 595 mg* (potassium gluconate 99 mg/caplet, 1–3/day) Dist: Rexall Sundown, Inc.	approved	✔	✔
🍁 Swiss™ Natural Sources Complex Potassium 50 mg (potassium proteinate complex 50 mg/caplet, 1/day) Dist: Swiss Herbal Remedies Ltd.	approved	✔	✔
The Medicine Shoppe® Natural Potassium 99 mg (potassium gluconate 99 mg/ caplet, 1/day) Dist: Medicine Shoppe International, Inc.	approved	✔	✔

Product (label info.)	Test Results		
	Approval	Contained labeled	Acceptable level
Thompson® Potassium 99 mg (potassium amino acid complex 99 mg/tablet, 1–3/day) Mf: Nutraceutical Corp.	approved	✔	✔
Trader Darwin's™ Potassium (potassium chloride 99 mg/tablet, 1/day) Dist: Trader Joe's	approved	✔	✔
Vitamin World® Naturally Inspired™ Potassium Citrate* (potassium citrate 99 mg/tablet, 1/day) Mf: Vitamin World, Inc.	approved	✔	✔
Vitasmart® Natural Potassium 99 mg (potassium gluconate 99 mg/caplet, 1/day) Dist: Kmart Corporation	approved	✔	✔
Winn-Dixie Natural Potassium 99 mg USP (potassium gluconate 99 mg/caplet, 1/day) Dist: Winn-Dixie Stores Inc.	approved	✔	✔

*Tested through CL's Voluntary Certification Program before, at the time of, or after the initial review.

✔ Check indicates the results met the criteria listed in the column heading.

‡ See also "More Brand Information," page 675.

🍁 Purchased from a retailer in Canada

Vitamin C

Vitamin C (ascorbic acid or dehydroascorbic acid) is an essential water-soluble vitamin that the human body can't manufacture. It must, therefore, come from foods or supplements. Fruits and vegetables are the richest food sources of vitamin C. Dietary supplements are typically sold as ascorbic acid, calcium ascorbate (Ester-C®), sodium ascorbate, or a combination of these forms. Supplements also commonly contain natural sources of vitamin C such as rose hips (the pear-shaped fruit of the rose, without the flower's petals) or acerola (a cherry-like fruit). (See ConsumerTips™ for Buying and Using, page 413.)

Vitamin C helps your body produce collagen, a basic component of connective tissue. Collagen is an important structural element in blood vessel walls, gums, and bones, making it particularly important to anyone recovering from wounds or surgery. Vitamin C also acts as an antioxidant, scavenging potentially harmful molecules called free radicals. Although not established by clinical trials, this antioxidant activity is theorized to help protect against cancer, cataracts, age-related macular degeneration of the retina, age-related skin changes and other chronic diseases. Vitamin C intake may be particularly helpful to smokers, who may suffer from oxidative stress and cell damage, which can deplete the body's store of vitamin C. Additionally, vitamin C supplements may boost the immune system under certain conditions, such as the period following endurance exercise. Vitamin C also enhances iron absorption from supplements and plant foods. However, vitamin C can also affect drugs you may be taking (see Concerns and Cautions, page 414).

Good sources of vitamin C include many vegetables, such as broccoli and brussel sprouts, as well citrus and other fruits. A healthful diet should provide the Recommended Dietary Allowance (RDA). (See ConsumerTips™ for Buying and Using, page 413.)

Quality Concerns and Product Testing

Regulations from the U.S. Food and Drug Administration (FDA) require that any vitamin C sold as a dietary supplement in the United States contain at least 100% of its labeled amount. The United States Pharmacopeia (USP) requires that products contain 100% to 120% of the claimed amount and that they meet certain specifications for disintegration and purity. Unfortunately, the FDA doesn't test for quality before sales, and products stating that they meet the USP standards don't always do so.

ConsumerLab.com tested several leading vitamin C dietary supplements to determine whether they contained 100% of the labeled amounts of vitamin C and whether tablets could break apart properly for absorption.

Test Findings

ConsumerLab.com purchased 29 brands of vitamin C–containing products: 27 for adults and 2 for children. All were tested for their levels of vitamin C. In addition, tablets and caplets were tested for their ability to disintegrate in simulated gastric fluid, as needed for absorption. (See the appropriate section in "ConsumerLab.com's Testing Methods and Standards," page 659, for more information.)

All of the 29 products tested met their claims for vitamin C and all applicable pill forms could disintegrate properly for absorption. Results were similarly positive in ConsumerLab.com's last review of vitamin C in 2003, although in 2001 several products were found to contain somewhat less vitamin C than claimed and one product would not disintegrate properly.

The 17 products that were selected for testing and a summary of the results are listed alphabetically in Test Results for Vitamin C Supplements. Also included in the list are 12 other products (indicated with an asterisk) that have met the same criteria through CL's Voluntary Certification Program (see Selection and Testing, page 25, volume 1).

ConsumerTips™ for Buying and Using

Both natural and synthetic vitamin C are equally recognized and used by your body, so all-natural rose-hip or acerola products provide no added benefit. In fact, some products stating "with rose hips," but not indicating the amount, may contain far more synthetic vitamin C than vitamin C from rose hips. Hint: A product's ingredient list gives a clue to the amount of rose hips present. Ingredients on that list must appear in the order of amount, from greatest to least. If rose hips appear last, the product has little.

Ester-C® (calcium ascorbate) is a nonacidic form of vitamin C that may be beneficial for people who experience symptoms of acid stomach from ordinary vitamin C. Note, however, that diarrhea associated with higher intakes of vitamin C has nothing to do with acidity. Ester-C® is also sometimes claimed to be better absorbed than regular ascorbic acid, but this claim has not been supported yet by reliable evidence.

Sodium ascorbate is also nonacidic. Products containing sodium ascorbate combined with ascorbic acid offer reduced acidity and are sometimes called "buffered vitamin C." Slow-release products may also help reduce digestive problems occurring with very high doses.

Some products claim "L-ascorbic acid"; it is just another name for vitamin C.

When looking for a dosage, remember that 1,000 mcg (micrograms) equals 1 mg (milligram), and 1,000 mg equals 1 gram. The Recommended Dietary Intake (RDA) is 90 mg a day for adult males and 75 mg a day for adult females. An additional 35 mg a day is recommended for smokers. For pregnant women younger than age 18, the RDA is 80 mg a day, and for pregnant women older than age 18, it's 85 mg/day. For breast-feeding women under age 18, the RDA is 115 mg a day, and for breast-feeding women older than age 18, it's 120 mg a day.

The RDA for children are as follows: 15 mg a day for children ages 1 to 3, 25 mg a day for children ages 4 to 8, and 45 mg a day for children ages 9 to 13. For males ages 14 to 18, the RDA is 75 mg a day. For females ages 14 to 18, it's 65 mg a day.

The RDA is achievable with healthful diets and is also more than adequate for normal collagen production. However, some healthcare professionals recommend higher daily doses of vitamin C, such as 500 to 1,500 mg/day for adults, claiming that such doses stimulate the immune system and help prevent some chronic diseases.

Vitamin C is safe when taken in moderate amounts, but too much vitamin C can cause diarrhea and other gastric disturbances. The Upper Tolerable Intake Level (UL, a dosage considered safe for most healthy adults) for vitamin C is 2,000 milligrams a day. For children, the UL intake is 400 mg a day for children ages 1 to 3, 650 mg a day for children ages 4 to 8, 1,200 mg a day for children ages 9 to 13, 1,800 mg a day for teens ages 14 to 18, and 2,000 mg a day for individuals ages 19 and older. Individuals are generally advised not to exceed these levels unless under medical supervision.

Concerns and Cautions

Long-term vitamin C treatment may increase the risk of kidney stones. However, evidence from large epidemiological studies indicates that people who regularly consume large amounts of vitamin C either experience no increased rate of kidney stone formation or actual protection from kidney stones. Nevertheless, case reports suggest that some individuals may be at increased risk for developing kidney stones if they take vitamin C supplements. For this reason, people with a history of kidney stones, or those with known defects in metabolism of oxalate or vitamin C, should probably limit vitamin C intake to RDA levels.

Another study has suggested that vitamin C might reduce the effectiveness of statin-type cholesterol-lowering drugs; however, this result has not been conclusively demonstrated.

And additional study suggests that high-dose vitamin C might reduce the effectiveness of the HIV drug indinavir.

Vitamin C may also interfere with the absorption of tricyclic antidepressants and anticoagulants.

Excess vitamin C from supplements can interfere with diagnostic tests for cholesterol, blood sugar levels, and blood in the stool.

The risk of liver damage from high doses of acetaminophen (Tylenol®) may be increased if you also take large doses (3 grams) of vitamin C.

Moreover, because vitamin C improves iron absorption, people with diseases that cause them to store too much iron should use vitamin C with caution.

Test-tube evidence suggests that vitamin C can cause the production of DNA-damaging genotoxins that may promote the development of cancer, an argument against high-dose vitamin C as a way to reduce cancer risk.

And one study found that taking vitamin C along with Pycnogenol (an extract of pine bark, also known as OPCs or oligomeric proanthocyanidins) might raise blood pressure levels in people with hypertension. The reasons for this unexpected finding are unclear.

Test Results for Vitamin C Supplements

Product (label info: amount of vitamin C/ pill type or other form, dosing)‡ Manufacturer (Mf) or Distributor (Dist)	Test Results	
	Approved or not approved	Broke apart properly
Children's		
ChildLife™ Essentials, Nutrition for Kids!™ Liquid Vitamin C (250 mg/5mL, 0.25–2/day) Dist: BioZeal	approved[1]	N/A
HealthAsure® Bear Essentials® Children's Vitamin C Gummi Bears (12 mg/gummi bear, 5/day) Dist: Health Asure, Inc.	approved	N/A
Adults/General: Vitamin C		
CVS® Pharmacy Vitamin C 500 mg USP (500 mg/ tablet, 1/day)* Dist: CVS Pharmacy, Inc.	approved	✔
Eckerd® Natural Vitamin C, 500 mg with rose hips, USP (500 mg/tablet, 1/day) Dist: Eckerd Drug Company	approved	✔
Member's Mark® Vitamin C 500 mg, Natural with Rose Hips, USP (500 mg/tablet, 1/day) Dist: Sam's West, Inc.	approved	✔

Product (label info.)	Test Results	
	Approval	**Broke apart**
Nature Made® C Vitamin 1,000 mg; Dietary Supplement USP Verified™ (1,000 mg/tablet, 1/day)* Dist: Nature Made Nutritional Products	approved	✔
Puritan's Pride® Time Release C-Time 500™ with Rose Hips (500 mg/tablet, 1/day)* Mf: Puritan's Pride, Inc.	approved	✔
Spring Valley® Ester-C® 500 mg (500 mg/tablet, 2/day)* Mf: Nature's Bounty	approved	✔
Sundown® Benefits C 1000 mg (1000 mg/caplet, 1/day)* Dist: Rexall Sundown, Inc	approved	✔
🍁 Swiss™ Natural Sources Timed Release Vitamin C 1,000 mg USP (1,000 mg/caplet, 1/day) Dist: Swiss Herbal Remedies Ltd.	approved	N/A
Vitamin World® Naturally Inspired™ Vitamin C-1,000 mg With Rose Hips, USP (1,000 mg/tablet, 1/day)* Mf: Vitamin World, Inc.	approved	✔

continued

417

Product (label info.)	Test Results	
	Approval	Broke apart
Vitamin World® Naturally Inspired™ Vitamin C-500 mg With Rose Hips, USP (500 mg/tablet, 1/day)* Mf: Vitamin World, Inc.	approved	✔
Vita-Smart® Natural Vitamin C 500 mg (500 mg/tablet, 1/day) Dist: Kmart Corporation	approved	✔
Adults/General: Vitamin C with Other Ingredients		
Country Life® Vegetarian Time Release Buffered Vitamin C, 500 mg Plus 100 mg of Bioflavonoids (500 mg/tablet, 1/day) Dist: Country Life	approved	N/A
Emer-gen-C® 1,000 mg of Vitamin C as Seven Mineral Asorbates, Lemon-Lime Fizzing Drink Mix (1,000 mg/package, 2/day) Dist: Alacer Corp.	approved[2]	N/A
Gary Null's Suprema C, Highly Absorbable Ascorbated Minerals, Buffered, Cherry (500 mg/chewable tablet, 1–3/day) Dist: Gary Null & Associates	approved	N/A

Product (label info.)	Test Results	
	Approval	**Broke apart**
LifeTime® Timed Release C-Complex, with Rose Hips, Bioflavonoids Rutin & Hesperidin (1,000 mg/ tablet, 1/day) Dist: LifeTime® Nutritional Specialties, Inc.	approved	N/A
Maxi-Health® Research Inc., Max-C 500™ (500 mg/ tablet, 1/day) Dist: Maxi-Health Research Inc.	approved	✔
Nature's Answer® Ester-C® with Bioflavonoids & Rose Hips (250 mg/capsule, 3/day) Dist: Nature's Answer	approved	N/A
Nature's Bounty® Ester-C® 1,000 mg, Non-Acidic Stomach Friendly, Coated for easy Swallowing (1,000 mg/tablet, 1/day)* Mf: Nature's Bounty, Inc.	approved	✔
Now® Chewable Ester-C® 500 mg, Great Orange Flavor (500 mg/lozenge, 1–3/day) Mf: Now Foods	approved	N/A
Nutrilite® Bio C Plus (250 mg/tablet, 1–4/day)* Dist: Access Business Group International LLC	approved	✔

continued

Product (label info.)	Test Results	
	Approval	Broke apart
🏃 Pharmanex® LifePak® Dietary Supplement, New! Anti-Aging Formula (250 mg calcium ascorbate/ packet, 2/day)* Dist: Pharmanex, LLC	approved; also approved for Alpha-Lipoic Acid, B Vitamins, Multivitamins, and Vitamin E	N/A
Pioneer® Vegetarian Vitamin C Complex, 500 mg, Naturally Buffered Indian Gooseberry & Bioflavonoids (500 mg/capsule, 3–6/day) Dist: Pioneer Nutritional Formulas, Inc.	approved[3]	N/A
Prairie Naturals® C-Force Plus, Mineral Ascorbates with Bioflavonoids (750 mg/ capsule, 1/day) Dist: Prairie Naturals®	approved	N/A
Puritan's Pride® Super C-500 Complex™ (500 mg/ tablet, 1/day)* Mf: Puritan's Pride, Inc.	approved	✔
Shaklee® Chewable Vita-C® 100 mg (100 mg/chewable tablet, 1/day) Dist: Shaklee Corporation	approved	N/A
Thompson® C 1,000 mg plus bioflavonoids (1,000 mg/capsule, 1/day) Mf: Nutraceutical Corp.	approved	N/A

Product (label info.)	Test Results	
	Approval	Broke apart
Vitamin World® Naturally Inspired™ Ester-C 500 mg With Bioflavonoids (500 mg/capsule, 2/day)* Mf: Vitamin World, Inc.	approved	N/A

N/A—Not applicable: Disintegration test applies only to tablets and caplets. Not applicable to chewable products, powders, capsules, liquid, and time-release forms.

‡ See also "More Brand Information," page 675.

* Tested through CL's Voluntary Certification Program before, at the time of, or after the initial review.

♦ Purchased from a retailer in Canada.

🏃 Product passed optional Athletic Banned Screening Program

[1] Maximum suggested serving size exceeds Upper Tolerable Intake Level (UL) for vitamin C for children under age 4.

[2] Suggested serving size exceeds UL for vitamin C for individuals under age 19.

[3] Serving of 3 capsules exceeds UL for vitamin C for individuals under age 19. Serving of 4 capsules exceeds UL for all adults.

Vitamin E Supplements and Skin Care Products

Vitamin E (alpha-tocopherol) is an antioxidant that assists in maintaining cell integrity. Only a relatively small amount of vitamin E is required to meet normal daily requirements. Though current recommended intakes can be easily obtained from foods, such as sunflower oil, safflower oil, canola oil, olive oil, many grains, nuts, and fruits, as well as fatty parts of meats, dietary surveys show that the majority of men and women in the United States fail to meet these recommendations for vitamin E. However, serious vitamin E deficiencies are rare in the United States.

Research using doses of vitamin E far higher than the recommended dietary intakes has provided evidence that it may be helpful for preventing preeclampsia and treating such diverse conditions as menstrual pain, tardive dyskinesia, cardiac autonomic neuropathy (a complication of diabetes), low sperm count, restless leg syndrome, acute anterior uveitis (inflammation of eye tissues), Alzheimer's disease, Parkinson's disease, and rheumatoid arthritis, among other conditions. Vitamin E might also improve seniors' immune response as measured by a variety of immune system markers. However, the evidence for its effectiveness in treating or preventing most of these conditions is inconclusive and research continues. (See ConsumerTips™ for Buying and Using, page 425.)

Vitamin E was long touted for preventing cardiovascular disease, but most of the recent studies have failed to prove vitamin E's effectiveness. However, many of these studies looked only at people already at high risk for heart disease or with a prior history of the condition. The initial studies that generated so much interest in vitamin E were population studies that, by definition, included a cross section of the population—some healthy people and some at high risk for heart disease. Some researchers have suggested that if vitamin E has any preventive powers against heart disease, it may be only in the earliest stages, before the damage is diagnosed. One study has even suggested that vitamin E supplements could, in fact, be harmful for some heart disease patients because the supplements could reduce the effectiveness of cholesterol-lowering agents. Although vitamin E was also once considered a promising treatment for preventing several kinds of cancer, current evidence points only to the prevention of prostate cancer. The National Cancer Institute is currently conducting a cancer prevention trial using a combination of the mineral selenium and vitamin E.

A recent analysis of data from several clinical trials suggests that high-dose vitamin E (in excess of 400 IU per day) may actually raise the risk of death slightly in older individuals with existing medical conditions.

Application of topical creams or gels containing vitamin E (usually as vitamin E acetate) in combination with melatonin or vitamin C have shown a bit of promise for helping to prevent sunburn; however, the effect is slight at best, and far less than that of standard sunblock. Weak preliminary evidence also hints that topical vitamin E might benefit blood circulation in people with diabetes. Vitamin E cream does not appear to help prevent surgical scarring.

Natural vs. Synthetic: Vitamin E is not one single molecule but a family of related molecules called tocopherols. There are several types of tocopherols, of which alpha-tocopherol is known to be the most biologically active. Alpha-tocopherol itself can exist in eight different forms, but only half of these forms are known to be useful in the body.

Natural vitamin E contains alpha-tocopherol exclusively in an active form, either as d-alpha-tocopherol or stabilized as d-alpha-tocopheryl acid succinate or d-alpha-tocopheryl acetate. Synthetic vitamin E (sometimes referred to as dl-alpha-tocopherol) contains both active and inactive forms of alpha-tocopherol. Natural vitamin E may also contain other types of tocopherols, such as beta-tocopherol, delta-tocopherol, and gamma-tocopherol. Some manufacturers use the term "mixed" tocopherols when referring to these different types. There are studies under way to determine whether gamma-tocopherol (which is more abundant in the diet than alpha-tocopherol) may be important for some of the beneficial effects associated with dietary vitamin E. At present, though, there is no hard evidence for this hypothesis. Note: Use of supplements containing high-dose alpha-tocopherol alone may decrease body levels of gamma- and delta-tocopherol. The implications of this information are unclear, but reduced levels of these natural tocopherols could be unhealthy.

The Recommended Dietary Allowance (RDA) for vitamin E is based only on active alpha-tocopherol. Consequently the amount of vitamin E needed by individuals to meet the RDA is different for natural versus synthetic vitamin E. In addition, too much vitamin E may cause bleeding resulting in hemorrhaging; therefore, Tolerable

Upper Intake Levels (UL) have been established to define safe vitamin E intake. (See ConsumerTips™ for Buying and Using.)

Quality Concerns and Product Testing

Neither the U.S. government nor any other agency is responsible for routinely testing vitamin E supplements or other dietary supplements for their contents or quality.

ConsumerLab.com, as part of its mission to independently evaluate products that affect health, wellness, and nutrition, purchased many of the leading vitamin E products sold in the U.S. and tested them for their quality.

Test Findings

Four vitamin E products failed to pass testing for having either too little vitamin E or for being synthetic when claiming to be natural. These four products were among 15 that ConsumerLab.com selected for testing. (See the appropriate section in "ConsumerLab.com's Testing Methods and Standards," page 660, in the appendix for more information.) These are the finding specifics:

Oral Supplements: Pure Encapsulations® Natural Vitamin E (with mixed tocopherols) contained some synthetic vitamin E despite labeling indicating only the natural form. Nature's Best Vitamin E-400 IU contained only 75% of its vitamin E despite claiming to be manufactured in accordance with "Good Manufacturing Practices" with "extensive quality control procedures to ensure . . . potency."

Creams and Oils: Derma-E® Vitamin E 12,000 IU Crème, Deep Moisturizing Formula contained only 58% of its expected amount of vitamin E. Jason® Pure, Natural & Organic Vitamin E Oil 5000 I.U. contained only 64% of its vitamin E, consisting primarily of synthetic vitamin E, despite claiming "pure, natural vitamin E." In addition, St. Ives Vitamin E Lotion claimed to contain vitamin E but did not specify an amount. This lack of information is typical with skin care products. CL found that the St. Ives product contained approximately 5 IU per mL, while the other topical products tested contained roughly 8 to 180 times that concentration.

The 15 products that were selected for testing and a summary of the results are listed alphabetically in Test Results for Vitamin E Supplements and Skin Care Products. Also included in the list are 19 other products (indicated with an asterisk) that have met the same criteria through CL's Voluntary Certification Program (see Selection and Testing, page 25, volume 1).

To help you compare products, the concentration of vitamin E in the creams and oils are shown in terms of IU per mL (milliliter). A teaspoon holds about 5 mL (4.93 mL), and one mL of oil or cream weighs about one gram.

ConsumerTips™ for Buying and Using

Natural and synthetic vitamin E in the proper doses can be equally active. However, it takes more IU of synthetic vitamin E than natural vitamin E to get the equivalent amount of active vitamin E, but it takes fewer IU of synthetic vitamin E than natural vitamin E to cause potential bleeding problems when high doses are used. IU on labels refer only to the amount of alpha and not to the other forms such as beta, gamma, and delta.

Products that may appear to be natural may not be. One important way to check is to look at the chemical name for vitamin E listed on the ingredient label. Natural vitamin E may be referred to as *d-alpha-tocopherol* or *mixed tocopherols* but should not include *dl-alpha-tocopherol* (which refers to synthetic vitamin E). Acceptable variations in the chemical names listed for natural vitamin E may include *tocopheryl* instead of *tocopherol* and may be followed by the words *acetate, succinate,* or *acid succinate.*

RDA: The Recommended Dietary Allowance (RDA) for vitamin E is based on milligrams of active alpha-tocopherol. However, most supplements are still labeled using IU and not milligrams. Complicating matters a bit, the conversion factor between IU and milligrams differs for natural vitamin E versus synthetic vitamin E. One IU of synthetic vitamin E equals 0.45 mg of active alpha-tocopherol, while one IU natural vitamin E equals 0.67 mg of active alpha-tocopherol.

Based on these conversion rates, the RDA for vitamin E as active alpha-tocopherol for children ages 1 to 3 is 6 mg a day (13 IU synthetic or 9 IU natural); for those ages 4 to 8, it is 7 mg a day (16 IU synthetic or 10 IU natural); and for those ages 9 to 13, it is 11 mg a day (24 IU synthetic or 16 IU natural). The RDA for individuals ages 14 and older is 15 mg a day (33 IU synthetic or 22 IU natural). However, the RDA for lactating women is 19 mg a day (42 IU synthetic or 28 IU natural).

UL: Some healthcare practitioners suggest doses generally much higher than the RDA for certain therapeutic or preventive uses. However, too much vitamin E may potentially cause bleeding that leads to hemorrhaging. Consequently, Tolerable Upper Intake Levels (UL) have been established for vitamin E from supplements and fortified foods and represent the highest daily intake that is unlikely to pose an adverse health risk. Any product that was tested for this review and exceeds the UL is indicated with a footnote.

As intake increases above the UL, the risk of adverse effects may increase, so you should not regularly exceed the UL unless the dosage is medically recommended and supervised. Because both the active and inactive forms of alpha-tocopherol found in synthetic vitamin E may contribute to bleeding, the UL for synthetic vitamin E are lower than those for natural.

The UL, therefore, translate approximately into these amounts per day: for children ages 1 to 3, the UL is 200 mg a day (220 IU synthetic or 300 IU natural); for those ages 4 to 8, it is 300 mg a day (330 IU synthetic or 450 IU natural); for those ages 9 to 13, it is 600 mg a day (660 IU synthetic or 900 IU natural); for those ages 14 to 18, it is 800 mg a day (880 IU synthetic or 1,200 IU natural); and for those ages 19 and older, it is 1,000 mg/day (1,100 IU synthetic or 1,500 IU natural). Unfortunately, if a natural vitamin E product is incorrectly labeled and actually made from synthetic vitamin E, even the most sophisticated users taking very high doses of vitamin E could accidentally find themselves exceeding the upper level.

Some researchers now think that the UL for vitamin E should be lowered, at least for certain groups of people. The reason is a study published in November 2004 that reanalyzed data from a large number of clinical studies involving vitamin E. The analysis showed a slight increase in the risk of death among older individuals with existing medical conditions using more than 400 IU of vitamin E per day. An increased risk of death was not seen at lower doses, and it is not known whether this risk would apply to younger or healthier individuals.

Special Uses: When vitamin E is used in a high dose to treat or prevent medical conditions, the dose used in studies has ranged widely, from 100 IU daily to 2000 IU daily. For most conditions, a dose of 100–600 IU daily has shown the most promise, though results are inconsistent, and in some cases, higher dosages seemed less effective than lower doses. For Alzheimer's disease, a dosage of 2000 IU daily has been tried with some success; for rheumatoid arthritis, a dosage of 600 IU twice daily has shown promise. NOTE: use of dosages above the UL is potentially dangerous and should be attempted only under physician supervision.

Topical Dosage: A variety of topical products containing vitamin E (or vitamin E acetate) in concentrations ranging from 2% to 100% have been used in preliminary studies. There is no clear evidence that more concentrated products are more effective than more dilute products.

When comparing the costs of vitamin E products, consider the dosage and the number of pills per bottle. Natural vitamin E generally costs a bit more for an equivalent amount of IU, but the cost may even out when converting doses into milligrams. If buying a vitamin E cream, you should expect the product to state its amount of vitamin E. Many do not.

Concerns and Cautions

Individuals who are on anticoagulant therapy, such as coumadin, or who are vitamin K deficient should be monitored by a physician when taking vitamin E supplements. Also potentially risky is combining high doses of vitamin E and aspirin or other agents that decrease platelet activity; take under a physician's care only.

Use of antioxidants such as vitamin E during cancer chemotherapy may be helpful in some circumstances and harmful in others. Always consult your physician before taking high dose vitamin E while undergoing cancer chemotherapy.

Test Results for Vitamin E Supplements and Skin Care Products

Product (label info: type and amount of vitamin E/unit, dosing)‡ Manufacturer (Mf) or distributor (Dist)	Claimed amount of vitamin E/unit and natural (N) or synthetic (S) form	Test Results		
		Approved or not approved	Contained claimed amount of vitamin E	Contained claimed form of vitamin E
Natural Vitamin E Supplements				
Carlson E-GEMS® Natural Vitamin E 400 IU (400 IU d-alpha tocopheryl acetate/softgel, 1/day)* Dist: Carlson Division of J.R. Carlson Laboratories Inc	400 IU (N)	approved	✔	✔
CVS® Pharmacy Natural Vitamin E 400 IU (USP) (400 IU d-alpha tocopheryl acetate/softgel, 1/day)* Dist: CVS Pharmacy, Inc.	400 IU (N)	approved	✔	✔
MaxiHealth® Circu-E 400™ (400 IU d-alpha tocopheryl succinate/ vegicap, 1–2/day) Dist: MaxiHealth Research Inc	400 IU (N)	approved	✔	✔

Product (label info.)	Claimed amount	Test Results		
		Approval	Contained claimed amount	Contained claimed form
Member's Mark® Natural d-Alpha E-400IU USP (400 IU d-alpha tocopheryl acetate/softgel, 1/day)[1] Dist: SWC	400 IU (N)	approved	✔	✔
Nutrilite® Parselenium-E® (400 IU vitamin E succinate/tablet, 1/day)* Dist: Access Business Group International LLC	400 IU (N)	approved	✔	✔
🏃 Pharmanex® LifePak® Dietary Supplement, New! Anti-Aging formula (150 IU d-alpha tocopheryl acetate/packet, 2/day)* Dist: Pharmanex, LLC	150 IU (N)	approved; also approved for alpha-lipoic acid, B vitamins, multi-vitamins, and vitamin C	✔	✔
Pure Encapsulations® Natural Vitamin E (with mixed tocopherols) (400 IU d-alpha tocopherol/ softgel, 1–2/day) Mf: Pure Encapsulations Inc	400 IU (N)	*not approved*	✔	Claims natural but contains some synthetic vitamin E.

continued

429

Product (label info.)	Claimed amount	Test Results		
		Approval	Contained claimed amount	Contained claimed form
Puritan's Pride® Natural Vitamin E 400 IU (d-Alpha, d-Beta, d-Gamma, d-Delta Tocopherols) (400 IU d-alpha, d-beta, d-gamma and d-delta tocopherols/ softgel, 1/day)* Mf: Puritan's Pride Inc	400 IU (N)	approved	✔	✔
Schiff® Cardio Care Natural Vitamin E Complex (400 IU D-alpha tocopherol, D-delta, D-beta and D-gamma tocopherol/ softgel, 1/day) Dist: Schiff® Products	400 IU (N)	approved	✔	✔
Shaklee® 400 IU Natural Vitamin E Plus Selenium, Vita-E® (400 IU d-alpha tocopheryl acid succinate/tablet, 1/day) Dist: Shaklee Corporation	400 IU (N)	approved	✔	✔

Product (label info.)	Claimed amount	Test Results		
		Approval	Contained claimed amount	Contained claimed form
Solgar® Natural Vitamin E 400 IU(400 IU d-alpha tocopherol/ softgel, 1/day)* Mf: Solgar Vitamin and Herb	400 IU (N)	approved	✔	✔
Spring Valley® Natural Vitamin E 400 IU d-alpha (400 IU d-alpha tocopherol/softgel, 1–3/day)* Dist: Rexall Sundown, Inc	400 IU (N)	approved	✔	✔
Sundown® Benefits Natural E 400 IU (400 IU d-alpha tocopherol/softgel, 1–3/day)* Dist: Rexall Sundown, Inc	400 IU (N)	approved	✔	✔
Vitamin World® Naturally Inspired™ 100% Natural E-400 IU USP d-alpha tocopheryl (400 IU d-alpha tocopheryl acetate/softgel, 1/day)* Mf: Vitamin World, Inc	400 IU (N)	approved	✔	✔

continued

Product (label info.)	Claimed amount	Test Results		
		Approval	Contained claimed amount	Contained claimed form
Vitamin World® Naturally Inspired™ Natural Vitamin E 400 IU, (d-Alpha, d-Beta, d-Gamma, d-Delta Tocopherols) (400 IU d-alpha, d-beta, d-gamma and d-delta tocopherols/ softgel, 1/day)* Mf: Vitamin World, Inc	400 IU (N)	approved	✔	✔
Synthetic or Synthetic & Natural Supplements				
CVS® Pharmacy Water Solubilized Vitamin E 400 IU USP (400 IU dl-alpha tocopheryl acetate/softgel, 1/day)* Dist: CVS Pharmacy Inc	400 IU (S)	approved	✔	✔
Mason natural® Vitamin E, E-400 IU Mixed (400 IU dl-alpha and d-alpha tocopherols with beta, gamma, and delta/softgel, 1/day) Dist by Mason Vitamins Inc	400 IU (S/N)	approved	✔	✔

Product (label info.)	Claimed amount	Test Results		
		Approval	Contained claimed amount	Contained claimed form
Nature Made® Vitamin E 400 IU Supplement USP (400 IU dl-alpha tocopheryl acetate/softgel, 1–2/day)* Dist: Nature Made Nutritional Products	400 IU (S)	approved	✔	✔
Nature's Best® Vitamin E-400 IU (400 IU dl-alpha tocopheryl acetate/gelcap, 1/day) Dist: Nature's Best Inc	400 IU (S)	**not** approved	Contained 75% of claimed vitamin E	✔
Origin® Vitamin E USP 400 IU (400 IU dl-alpha tocopheryl acetate/softgel, 1/day)* Dist: Target Corporation	400 IU (S)	approved	✔	✔
PharmAssure™ Vitamin E 400 IU (400 IU dl-alpha tocopheryl acetate/softgel, 1/day) Dist: PharmAssure, Inc	400 IU (S)	approved	✔	✔

continued

433

Product (label info.)	Claimed amount	Test Results		
		Approval	Contained claimed amount	Contained claimed form
Puritan's Pride® Vitamin E-400 IU USP (400 IU dl-alpha tocopheryl acetate/softgel, 1/day)* Mf: Puritan's Pride, Inc	400 IU (S)	approved	✔	✔
Spring Valley® Vitamin E 1000 IU (in a water soluble base) USP (1000 IU dl-alpha tocopheryl acetate/softgel, 1/day)* Mf: Nature's Bounty, Inc	1000 IU (S)	approved	✔	✔
Sundown® Benefits E 400 IU (400 IU dl-alpha tocopheryl acetate/softgel, 1-3/day) * Dist: Rexall Sundown Inc	400 IU (S)	approved**	✔	✔
Vitamin World® Vitamin E-400 I.U. USP (400 IU dl-alpha tocopheryl acetate/softgel, 1/day)* Mf: Vitamin World Inc	400 IU (S)	approved	✔	✔

Product (label info.)	Claimed amount	Test Results		
		Approval	Contained claimed amount	Contained claimed form
Walgreens® Vitamin E 400 IU USP Dietary Supplement (400 IU dl-alpha tocopheryl acetate/softgel, 1/day) Dist: Walgreen Co.	400 IU (S)	approved	✔	✔
Windmill™ Vitamin E-200 (200 IU dl-alpha tocopheryl acetate/softgel, 1/day) Mf: Windmill Health Products	200 IU (S)	approved	✔	✔
Creams and Lotions				
Derma-E® Vitamin E 12,000 IU Crème, Deep Moisturizing Formula (106.2 IU tocopheryl acetate/1g cream, 2g/day) Dist: Derma-E Products	106.2 IU/g (Form not stated)	*not* approved	Contained 58% of claimed vitamin E	✔

continued

Product (label info.)	Claimed amount	Test Results		
		Approval	Contained claimed amount	Contained claimed form
St. Ives® Swiss Formula®, Advanced Therapy Lotion Vitamin E and Vitamin A (5 IU tocopheryl acetate/mL of cream, dose not stated) Mf: St. Ives Laboratories	Found to contain 5 IU/mL*** (Amount and form not stated)	N/A	✔	✔
Topical Oils				
Ethical Nutrients® Mycel® Vitamin E (150 IU d-alpha tocopheryl acetate/mL, 1 mL (20 drops/day) Dist: Ethical Nutrients	150 IU/mL (N)	approved	✔	✔
GNC Nourishskin™ Vitamin E Skin Oil (56,000 IU) 4.8 fl oz. (142mL) (394.4 IU tocopheryl acetate/mL, dose not stated) Dist: General Nutrition Corporation	394.4 IU/mL (Form not stated)	approved	✔	✔

Product (label info.)	Claimed amount	Test Results		
		Approval	Contained claimed amount	Contained claimed form
Jason® Pure, Natural & Organic Vitamin E Oil 5000 I.U. 95% Organic Pure Beauty Oil With 5 Exotic Oils (42.4 IU tocopheryl acetate/mL, dose not stated) Mf: Jason Natural Cosmetics	42.4 IU/ mL (N)	*not* approved	Had 64% of claimed vitamin E	Label suggests natural vitamin E; tests found mostly primarily synthetic
Puritan's Pride® Natural Vitamin E-Oil (30,000 IU) Vegetarian Formula 2.5 fl.oz (74mL)* (405.4 IU d-alpha tocopheryl acetate/mL, 0.25 mL (5 drops/day) Mf: Puritan's Pride Inc	405.4 IU/ mL (N)	approved	✔	✔
Vitamin World® Pure E-Oil 70,000 IU, 2.5 fl.oz (75mL)* (933 IU tocopheryl acetate/mL, dose not stated) Mf: Vitamin World Inc	933 IU/mL (Form not stated)	approved	✔	✔

continued

Product Reviews: Vitamins & Minerals

✔ Check indicates the results met the criteria listed in the column heading.

‡ See also "More Brand Information," page 675.

*Tested through CL's Voluntary Certification Program before, at the time of, or after the initial review.

**Exceeds tolerable upper intake level (UL) for adults for vitamin E.

***Amount found on testing—amount not stated on label.

🏃 Product passed optional Athletic Banned Screening Program

[1]The approval status of this product was updated on 10/24/04 based on additional scientific information.

Zinc Supplements (Lozenges, Pills, and Liquids)

Zinc is an essential mineral, one of the few nutrients for which a number of people are mildly deficient. Zinc deficiency is especially common in adolescents, infants, seniors, and women in general. Certain drugs and nutrients can inhibit zinc absorption and/or increase its excretion. Thus, for many people, increasing the intake of zinc-containing foods or taking a zinc supplement, either alone or as part of a multivitamin/multimineral, may be a prudent form of nutritional insurance.

As a dietary supplement, zinc is found in many forms, including zinc gluconate, zinc acetate, zinc citrate, zinc sulfate, zinc chelates, zinc carbonate, zinc orotate, and zinc picolinate. (See ConsumerTips™ for Buying and Using, page 441, for information about the forms of zinc and foods that contain zinc.)

Zinc plays a role in brain function, wound healing, and sperm production. Zinc in pill or liquid form may be taken in nutritional doses to replenish depleted zinc levels. Among people who are deficient in zinc (especially the elderly), some evidence suggests that such replenishment might help increase immunity.

As a lozenge or nasal gel, zinc may act directly in the throat or nose to reduce the duration of the common cold. NOTE: There have been unconfirmed reports of loss of smell resulting from zinc nasal gel. (For more information about ingredients used to treat or prevent colds see product reviews of Echinacea, page 238, volume 1; Vitamin C, page 412; and Asian and American Ginseng, page 225, volume 1.) Zinc syrup taken by mouth and swallowed may slightly help prevent and/or treat common colds in children.

Some people take zinc at higher-than-recommended nutritional levels for various purposes, including: slowing the progression of age-related macular degeneration; enhancing the effectiveness of antidepressants; reducing mouth and skin irritation during radiation therapy for head and neck cancer; improving symptoms of acne, anorexia nervosa, sickle cell anemia; altered taste sensation (of various origins); attention-deficit-hyperactivity disorder (ADHD); and peptic ulcers. However, the evidence that zinc at high dosage levels works for all of these purposes is incomplete at best. Furthermore, such high doses of zinc can have adverse effects. (See ConsumerTips™

for Buying and Using, page 441, for dosage and safety issues regarding zinc supplements.)

Quality Concerns and Product Testing

No government agency is responsible for routinely testing zinc or other dietary supplements for their contents or quality. ConsumerLab. com purchased and evaluated zinc supplements to determine whether they contained the amounts of the zinc stated on their labels. Products were also tested for lead, a potential contaminant in mineral supplements. All nonchewable tablets were also tested to be sure that they would properly disintegrate to enable their absorption. (See "ConsumerLab.com's Testing Methods and Standards," page 661.) Thirteen zinc supplements were tested. ConsumerLab.com selected nine. Four others (each indicated with an asterisk) were tested at the request of their manufacturers/distributors through CL's Voluntary Certification Program and are included for having passed testing. Also listed are two products similar to ones that passed but sold under different brand names.

Test Findings

Unlike results in 2003, when ConsumerLab.com found two zinc supplements to contain less ingredient than claimed (73% and 85%), recent tests found all selected products to meet their claims. All passed lead testing, and all tablets and caplets were able to properly break apart to release their ingredients.

Although all products passed quality testing, there are notable differences among them that should be considered:

Lozenges: Among the four lozenges, there was significant variation in the zinc per lozenge (from 5 mg to 13.3 mg) and the suggested daily serving. Only Cold-Eeze All Natural Cherry suggested a dosage known to be effective for reducing the severity and duration of cold symptoms—13.3 mg every 2 hours. The other three did not clearly state how often to take a lozenge: Runny Rhino Cold Relief Pops with Zinc advised "Repeat as necessary" but warned not to exceed eight pops per day. Sunkist Zinc Throat Lozenges suggested "2–8 times daily." And Zand Lemon Zinc Herbalozenge simply advised "May be repeated as needed."

Too much zinc over extended periods of time can cause problems. (See ConsumerTips™ for Buying and Using for information about dosage and safety issues.) But the lozenges from Sunkist and Zand suggested no limit on how long to use them. Better in this regard were warnings on Runny Rhino to discontinue if symptoms persist and Cold-Eeze, which suggested to consult a physician "if symptoms worsen, or persist beyond 7 days."

Pills and Liquids: The zinc pills and liquids generally provided 25 mg to 50 mg of zinc. These amounts are in the correct range for treating zinc deficiencies or providing high-dose zinc to treat or prevent various conditions (see ConsumerTips™ for Buying and Using section to follow).

ConsumerTips™ for Buying and Using

Food Sources: Oysters have very high zinc content (about 8 mg zinc per oyster). Other forms of shellfish, as well as organ meats, beef, pork, and chicken can provide 1 to 8 mg of elemental zinc per serving. Whole grains, legumes, nuts, and seeds provide zinc as well, ranging in amounts from 0.2 to about 3 mg per serving, but the high phytic acid (phytate) content of these foods may reduce the zinc's availability. Many breakfast cereals and nutrition bars are also fortified with zinc.

Supplements: Zinc supplements come in various forms, known as zinc salts or complexes. Zinc sulfate is the least expensive zinc salt, but zinc acetate, gluconate, citrate, or picolinate may be better absorbed. Note that there is a difference between the milligrams of pure zinc ("elemental zinc") in a product and the total amount of the zinc salt. In this article and product list, we use numbers based on the elemental zinc itself, not the salt.

To Prevent or Treat Deficiency: Mild zinc deficiency is fairly common. The Recommended Dietary Allowance (RDA) of zinc is 3 mg for children ages 1 to 3, 5 mg for those 4 to 8, and 8 mg for those 9 to 13. For males 14 and older, the RDA is 11 mg. For females 14 to 18, it is 9 mg, while for those 19 years and older, it is 8 mg per day. The RDA for pregnant women who are 18 years or younger is 13 mg, while it is 11 mg for pregnant women 19 years and older. For lactating women the RDAs are 14 mg if 18 years or younger, or 12 mg if 19 years or older. High-fiber foods may interfere with zinc supplement absorption if the foods and the supplement are taken at the same time. Certain drugs may increase the need for zinc supplements, such as ACE inhibitors, thiazide diuretics, and medications that reduce stomach acid (such as Prilosec or Pepcid).

To Shorten a Cold (Lozenges and Gels): Most but not all studies suggest that when zinc is taken in the form of a lozenge or nasal gel (as opposed to an oral supplement), it can directly kill cold viruses and thereby shorten the duration of a cold. Only zinc gluconate and zinc acetate have been shown to be effective for this purpose, although other forms of zinc are available on the market in lozenges. It is thought that certain flavorings that may be added to lozenges, such as citric acid and tartaric acid, can interfere with zinc's antiviral action. The flavorings (sweeteners) dextrose, sucrose, sorbitol, and mannitol are thought not to interfere. Products are available in which zinc is mixed with a great variety of other substances, such as herbs or vitamin C, but these have not been tested for their combined efficacy. Zinc sulfate syrup may help prevent colds in children, as well as reduce the duration and symptoms in kids who catch colds.

A typical dose of the lozenge form of zinc is 13 to 23 mg of zinc taken every 2 hours during the day. It is important not to take this much zinc for more than a week or so, as the amount greatly exceeds the tolerable intake levels discussed (see Concerns and Cautions). It is possible that concern over excess zinc is the reason that several products on the market suggest a dose of only one or two lozenges per day. However, zinc lozenges are not likely to help a cold if taken this way, so you may need to use these more frequently. Some people may get an upset stomach from the lozenges. Because zinc needs to act in the throat, let the lozenge dissolve fully—do not chew it or swallow it whole.

In children, zinc sulfate syrup in a dose of 15 mg of zinc per day may help prevent colds and 30 mg of zinc per day at the first onset of symptoms may help treat a cold, although the benefits appear to be modest. In the seven-month study from which these results were reported, side effects were minor and similar among the zinc-treated children and those treated with placebo (sugar pills). However, the children in the study were not monitored for signs of zinc overload or other potentially serious side effects of taking high doses of zinc for many months. Doses exceeding the UL for children should be used only under physician supervision.

To Prevent Macular Degeneration: A large study known as AREDS (Age-Related Eye Disease Study) looked at the effects of supplements on eye health. It found that zinc alone (80 mg) or with the antioxidants vitamin C (500 mg), vitamin E (400 IU), and beta-carotene (15 mg), could help prevent or slow the progression of age-related macular degeneration when taken on a daily basis.

(Participants were also given copper at 2 mg daily to help offset the reduced copper absorption caused by zinc—see Concerns and Cautions below.) Antioxidants alone were not particularly effective, but zinc alone did provide some significant benefits. This study failed to find benefits regarding the development or progression of cataracts.

Other compounds may improve eye health—see product review of lutein and zeaxanthin, page 193, volume 1.

Other Uses: Some evidence suggests that 30 mg of zinc taken orally each day may be helpful for acne. This is a safe dose for most people. However, in many studies of zinc for acne, a much higher dose was used: 90 mg daily or more. Doses this high should be used only under physician supervision (see Concerns and Cautions). Relatively high doses of zinc have also been recommended for other diseases, including anorexia nervosa, sickle cell anemia, altered taste sensation (of various origins), and attention-deficit/hyperactivity disorder. The balance of current evidence fails to support the use of zinc for cataracts, rheumatoid arthritis, or eczema. The use of zinc in high or low doses for benign prostatic hyperplasia (BPH), peptic ulcers, diabetes, male infertility, osteoporosis, Crohn's disease, tinnitus (ringing in the ear), mouth and skin irritation during radiation therapy for head and neck cancer, and many other conditions for which it is often recommended remains highly speculative.

Concerns and Cautions

Zinc supplements cause few immediate side effects other than occasional stomach upset or unpleasant taste. The established tolerable upper intake levels (UL) for daily intake (amounts that should be safe when taken long term by almost anyone who is in good health) for zinc are: 7 mg for children ages 1 to 3, 12 mg for those 4 to 8, 23 mg for those 9 to 13, 34 mg for those 14 to 18, and 40 mg for individuals 19 years and older.

Excessive intake of zinc can interfere with the absorption of copper, leading to copper deficiency. The combination of excess zinc and deficient copper can dangerously suppress the immune system and also cause anemia and heart problems. In order to partially offset these risks, it is generally considered advisable to take copper at a dose of 1–3 mg daily when taking zinc supplements long term.

As noted earlier, when using zinc lozenges for the treatment of the common cold, one is taking zinc at doses exceeding the UL. Such short-term use should be safe, but should be limited to no more than one to two weeks. Doses exceeding the UL for more than a week or two should be used only under physician supervision.

Long-term zinc supplementation at very high doses (over 100 mg per day) has been associated with an increased risk of prostate cancer. Zinc's overall role in prostate cancer, however, is unclear, as there is also research indicating that zinc may suppress prostate cancer cell growth.

Zinc nasal gel has been linked in reports to permanent or temporary loss of smell, as well as pain in the nose immediately after use.

Zinc can impair the absorption of antibiotics in the tetracycline or fluoroquinolone families (e.g., doxycycline, tetracycline, ciprofloxacin, Cipro, Noroxin), as well as the drug penicillamine. In addition, combined use of zinc supplements and the drug amiloride might lead to excess zinc in the body.

Test Results for Zinc Supplements

Product (label info: amount of elemental zinc [form] per unit, dose)‡ Daily amount of Mf suggested zinc Manufacturer (Mf) or Distributor (Dist)	Test Results			
	Approved or not approved	Contained claimed amount of zinc	Accept-able levels of lead***	Broke apart properly
Lozenges				
Cold-Eeze® Homeopathic, Cherry (13.3 mg zinc per lozenge, 6 lozenges/day) Daily: 79.8 mg[1] zinc gluconate Mf: The Quigley Corporation	approved	✔	✔	N/A
Runny Rhino Cold Relief Pops with Zinc®, Vitamin C (6.65 mg zinc per lozenge, up to 8 pops/day) Daily: 6.65 mg–53.2 mg[1] chelated zinc Dist: Improvita Health Products, Inc.	approved[2]	✔	✔	N/A

continued

Product (label info.)	Test Results			
	Approval	Contained claimed	Accept- able levels	Broke apart
Sunkist® Mixed Flavors Zinc Throat Lozenges, with Vitamin C and Echinacea (5 mg zinc from zinc citrate and gluconate per lozenge, 2–8 lozenges/day) Daily: 10–40 mg[1] from zinc citrate and gluconate Dist: WN Pharmaceuticals® Inc.	approved[2]	✔	✔	N/A
Zand® Lemon Zinc Herbalozenge® Natural Lemon Flavor (5 mg zinc [from zinc gluconate] per lozenge, may be repeated as needed) Daily: Unlimited[1] (zinc gluconate) Mf: Zand Herbal Formulas	approved[2]	✔	✔	N/A

Product (label info.)	Test Results			
	Approval	Contained claimed	Accept-able levels	Broke apart
Liquid and Pills				
Eckerd® Natural Zinc 50 mg (50 mg zinc per tablet, 1/day) Daily: 50 mg[1] zinc gluconate Dist: Eckerd Drug Company	approved	✔	✔	✔
Natural Factors® Zinc Chelate 25 mg (25 mg zinc per tablet, 1–2/day) Daily: 25–50 mg[1] HVP chelate Dist: Natural Factors	approved	✔	✔	✔
Nature Made® Zinc 30 mg (30 mg per tablet, 1/day) Daily: 30 mg zinc[1] Dist: Nature Made Nutritional products	approved	✔	✔	✔
NOW® Zinc 50 mg (50 mg zinc per tablet, 1/day) Daily: 50 mg[1] zinc gluconate Mf: NOW Foods	approved	✔	✔	✔

continued

Product (label info.)	Test Results			
	Approval	Contained claimed	Accept-able levels	Broke apart
Puritan's Pride® Chelated Zinc 25 mg (25 mg zinc per tablet, 1/day)* Daily: 25 mg[1] zinc gluconate Mf: Puritan's Pride, Inc	approved	✔	✔	✔
Puritan's Pride® Picolinate Zinc 25 mg (25 mg zinc per caplet, 1/day)* Daily: 25 mg[1] zinc picolinate Mf: Puritan's Pride, Inc	approved	✔	✔	✔
Thorne Research Zinc Citrate, Hypo-Allergenic (30 mg zinc [from zinc citrate] per capsule) Daily: Not specified[1] Mf: Thorne Research	approved	✔	✔	N/A

Product (label info.)	Test Results			
	Approval	Contained claimed	Accept-able levels	Broke apart
Trace Minerals Research Ionic Zinc 50 mg (50 mg zinc per 1.25 mL, 1.25 mL/day) Daily: 50 mg[1] zinc sulfate Dist: Trace Minerals Research	approved	✔	✔	N/A
Vitamin World® Naturally Inspired™ Chelated Zinc 50 mg (50 mg zinc per caplet, 1/day)* Daily: 50 mg[1] zinc gluconate Mf: Vitamin World, Inc	approved	✔	✔	✔

Similar to Approved Products:**

Puritan's Pride® Chelated Zinc 50 mg (50 mg zinc [from zinc gluconate] per caplet, 1/day)*

Mf: Puritan's Pride, Inc

Vitamin World® Naturally Inspired® Chelated Zinc 25 mg Zinc gluconate (25 mg zinc [from zinc gluconate] per tablet, 1/day)*

Mf: Vitamin World, Inc

‡ See also "More Brand Information," page 675.

*Tested through CL's Voluntary Certification Program prior to, at time of, or after initial posting of this Product Review.

continued

**Product identical in formulation and manufacture to a product that has passed testing but sold under a different brand. For more information on CL's Multi-Label Testing Program see Selection and Testing section, page 25, volume 1.

*** Limits: Lead—0.5 mcg per day;

[1] May exceed the Upper Tolerable Intake Level (UL) for specific age groups. ULs: 7 mg for children ages 1 to 3, 12 mg for those 4 to 8, 23 mg for those 9 to 13, 34 mg for those 14 to 18, and 40 mg for individuals 19 years and older (see Concerns and Cautions, page 443).

[2] Amount of elemental zinc per lozenge and suggested serving information is not consistent with products shown to shorten colds and decrease symptoms in adults (see ConsumerTips™ for Buying and Using, page 441).

✔ Check indicates the results met the criteria listed in the column heading.

N/A—Not applicable.

Part 5

Product Reviews:
Special Ingredients

Alpha-Lipoic Acid

Alpha-lipoic acid (or lipoic acid) is naturally produced in the body, assisting in the conversion of glucose to energy. It also acts as an antioxidant, able to neutralize harmful chemicals known as free radicals. It can function in both water and fat, as opposed to the antioxidants vitamin E (which works only in fat) and vitamin C (which works only in water). It may also be able to regenerate these other antioxidants after they have neutralized free radicals.

As an oral supplement alpha-lipoic acid seems to reduce symptoms of peripheral neuropathy in diabetes patients, improving symptoms such as burning, pain, numbness, and prickling of the feet and legs as well as improving sensation. There is evidence that alpha-lipoic acid supplements may also help diabetic patients by lessening damage of the heart, kidneys, and small blood vessels. Alpha-lipoic acid may also improve blood sugar control in people with type 2 diabetes, but it doesn't seem to lower glycosylated hemoglobin (HgbA1c) levels.

Alpha-lipoic acid may be helpful in treating burning mouth syndrome (BMS), a condition characterized by unexplained scalding sensations in the mouth. Preliminary studies suggest that it might also help prevent or treat a myriad of conditions including age-related hearing loss, glaucoma, cancer, and cataracts. Its antioxidant effects might provide protection in cerebral ischemia, other causes of damage to brain or neural tissue, mitochondrial dysfunction, liver disease, aminoglycoside-induced cochlear damage, heavy metal and chemical poisoning, and radiation exposure. Alpha-lipoic acid inhibits replication of the human immunodeficiency virus (HIV) in vitro and in AIDS patients might improve blood antioxidant status and increase T-helper lymphocytes and T-helper to T-helper suppressor cell ratio.

Quality Concerns and Product Testing

Prior studies by ConsumerLab.com found a small percentage of alpha-lipoic acid supplements to lack the full amount of this ingredient. In a group of 13 products tested in 2004, ConsumerLab.com found one with only 15% of its alpha-lipoic acid. In 2005, tests of nine Japanese products identified one that had no alpha-lipoic acid. Neither the FDA nor any other federal or state agency routinely tests alpha-lipoic acid supplements for quality prior to sale.

ConsumerLab.com, as part of its mission to independently evaluate products that affect health, wellness, and nutrition, purchased several dietary supplements sold in the U.S. claiming to contain alpha-lipoic acid. These were tested for their amount of alpha-lipoic acid and for potential lead contamination. Standard tablets and caplets were also tested for their ability to properly disintegrate ("break apart") as needed for absorption.

Test Findings

Tests showed that two of the 11 alpha-lipoic acid supplements that ConsumerLab.com chose to test contained significantly less ingredient than promised on their labels. Pro-Caps® Laboratories Andrew Lessman Alpha-lipoic Acid contained only 51% of its claimed amount. Among its ingredients was thiamin, which is known to degrade alpha-lipoic acid and may explain the low level found. Ironically, the label on this product touted unsurpassed quality and integrity. Thompson® Alpha-lipoic Acid 50 mg contained only 88% of its claimed amount. None of the products contained unacceptable levels of lead, nor failed to break apart properly, which is necessary for absorption. See "ConsumerLab.com's Testing Methods and Standards," page 662, for more information about how products were evaluated.

Listed alphabetically in Test Results for Alpha-Lipoic Acid Supplements are the 11 alpha-lipoic acid products selected by ConsumerLab.com and three others (each indicated with an asterisk) that passed the same evaluation through ConsumerLab.com's Voluntary Certification Program. Also listed are two products similar to ones that passed but sold under different brand names.

ConsumerTips™ for Buying and Using

Alpha-lipoic acid comes in a wide range of pill strengths. In this review, products ranged from 15 mg to 600 mg per pill. Choose a product that will allow you to conveniently get the dose that you intend to take (see Dosage information below). Be sure to know what dose is appropriate for you rather than relying on the label information. Manufacturers' suggested doses ranged from 50 mg to 1,200 mg per day.

Mixed vs. Natural Form: Clinical trials to date with alpha-lipoic acid used a form consisting of equal amounts of R (or D) and S (or L) isomers. This mixed (or "racemic") form is the most commonly available type on the market. Animal studies suggests that the R isomer (which is the naturally occurring form) may be more effective in improving insulin sensitivity than the S isomer, but clinical studies have not yet been conducted to judge the relative effectiveness and safety of this form in people. Products claiming to contain only the R isomer are available on the market and are generally more expensive than the mixed form. As of the time of this review, there was no published method and no chemical standard available for testing for the R form. R-only products were consequently not included in this Review but they may be tested in the future as the science evolves.

Dosage: Although a healthy body makes enough alpha-lipoic acid to supply its requirements, and you can get some alpha-lipoic acid from liver and yeast, supplementation is necessary to get therapeutic dosages. The typical dosage of oral alpha-lipoic acid for treating diabetes, peripheral neuropathy, and cardiac autonomic neuropathy is 600 to 1,200 mg per day divided into three equal doses. Several weeks of treatment are often necessary for full effects to develop. For peripheral neuropathy, there is some preliminary evidence that alpha-lipoic acid may be more effective if it is combined with GLA (gamma-linolenic acid), another supplement.

For use as a general antioxidant, a lower dosage of 20 to 50 mg daily is commonly recommended; although there is no evidence that taking alpha-lipoic acid in this way offers any health benefit.

Concerns and Cautions

Because alpha-lipoic acid may help control blood sugar in diabetics, adjustments may be needed to anti-diabetic medication when using alpha-lipoic acid.

Paresthesias (abnormal skin sensations) have been reported to worsen temporarily at the beginning of therapy.

Skin rash has been reported with use of alpha-lipoic acid.

Particularly at higher doses, alpha-lipoic acid can cause gastrointestinal upset, including nausea and vomiting, and headache, although these side effects are more common with higher doses and when given intravenously. Very large doses of alpha-lipoic acid have caused serious toxicity in thiamine-deficient animals. People taking high doses of alpha-lipoic acid who are at risk for thiamine deficiency, such as alcoholics, may require thiamine supplementation.

Test Results for Alpha-Lipoic Acid Supplements

Product (label info: amount of alpha-lipoic acid/ unit, dose)‡ Daily amount of alpha-lipoic acid (Mf suggested) Manufacturer (Mf) or Distributor (Dist)	Test Results		
	Approved or not approved	Contained claimed amount of alpha-lipoic acid	Purity from lead contamination
Age-Less Rx™ Sustained Release Alpha-lipoic Acid, 300 mg (300 mg/ tablet, 3–4/day) Daily: 900 mg– 1,200 mg Mf: Medical Research Institute	approved	✔	✔
Bronson Labs™ Alpha-lipoic Acid 100 mg (100 mg/ capsule, 2–3/day) Daily: 200 mg–300 mg Dist: Bronson Laboratories	approved	✔	✔

Product (label info.)	Test Results		
	Approval	Contained claimed	Purity from lead
Life Wise® Naturals Alpha-lipoic Acid 50 mg (50 mg/ capsule, 1–2/day) Daily: 50 mg–100 mg Dist: Life Wise Naturals, Inc	approved	✔	✔
Natural Factors® Alpha-Lipoic Acid 200 mg (200 mg/ capsule, 3/day) Daily: 600 mg Mf: Natural Factors	approved	✔	✔
Nature's Bounty® Alpha-lipoic Acid 100 mg (100 mg/ capsule, 1/day)* Daily: 100 mg Mf: Nature's Bounty, Inc	approved	✔	✔
Nature's Life® Alpha-lipoic Acid 200 mg (200 mg/ softgel, 1–3/day) Daily: 200 mg–600 mg Dist: Nature's Life	approved	✔	✔

continued

Product (label info.)	Test Results		
	Approval	Contained claimed	Purity from lead
Pharmanex® LifePak® Dietary Supplement, New! Anti-Aging Formula (15 mg/packet, 2/ day)* Daily: 30 mg Dist: Pharmanex, LLC	approved; also approved for B vitamins, multivitamins, vitamin C, and vitamin E	✔	✔
Pro-Caps® Laboratories Andrew Lessman Alpha-lipoic Acid, n-acetyl cysteine (100 mg/capsule, 1/day) Daily: 100 mg Mf: Pro-Caps Laboratories	*not* approved	Contained only 50.6% of claimed amount	✔
Pure Encapsulations® Alpha-lipoic Acid 600 mg (600 mg/ capsule, 1–2/day) Daily: 600 mg– 1,200 mg Mf: Pure Encapsulations, Inc.	approved	✔	✔

continued

Product (label info.)	Test Results		
	Approval	Contained claimed	Purity from lead
Puritan's Pride® Alpha-lipoic Acid 300 mg (300 mg/ softgel, 2/day)* Daily: 600 mg Mf: Puritan's Pride, Inc	approved	✔	✔
Solgar® Alpha-lipoic Acid 200 mg (200 mg/capsule, 1/day) Daily: 200 mg Mf: Solgar Vitamin and Herb	approved	✔	✔
Source Naturals® Alpha-lipoic Acid 300 mg (300 mg/ capsule, 1/day) Daily: 300 mg Dist: Source Naturals	approved	✔	✔
The Vitamin Shoppe® Antioxidants, Alpha-Lipoic Acid 300 mg (300 mg/ capsule, 1/day) Daily: 300 mg Dist: The Vitamin Shoppe®	approved	✔	✔

continued

Product Reviews: Special Ingredients

Product (label info.)	Test Results		
	Approval	**Contained claimed**	**Purity from lead**
Thompson® Alpha-lipoic Acid 50 mg (50 mg/tablet, 2/day) Daily: 100 mg Mf: Nutraceutical Corp. for Thompson Nutritionals, Inc	*not* approved	Contained only 88.2% of claimed amount	✔

Similar to Approved**

Puritan's Pride® Alpha-lipoic Acid 100 mg (100 mg/capsule, 1/day)

Dist: Puritan's Pride, Inc

Vitamin World® Naturally Inspired™ Alpha-lipoic Acid 100 mg (100 mg/capsule, 1/day)

Dist: Vitamin World, Inc

---

*Tested through CL's Voluntary Certification Program prior to, at time of, or after initial posting of this Product Review.

**Product identical in formulation and manufacture to a product that has passed testing but sold under a different brand. For more information on CL's Multi-Label Testing Program see Selection and Testing, page 25, volume 1.

‡ See also "More Brand Information," page 675.

CLA (Conjugated Linoleic Acid) for Slimming

CLA (conjugated linoleic acid) is a polyunsaturated fatty acid found naturally in milk and meat and produced from safflower and sunflower oils.

CLA may help with slimming by increasing the ratio of muscle to fat, that is, increasing lean body mass; it does not, however, reduce overall weight. (For weight-loss products, see " Weight-Loss Supplements: Bitter Orange, Green Tea, 7-Keto-DHEA, Pyruvate," page 202, volume 1.) And some studies indicate CLA might improve insulin levels in people with diabetes; however, other studies suggest that it is not a useful supplement for people with diabetes, and might, in fact, contribute to a prediabetic state in obese people. In animals and test tube studies, CLA has shown some ability to inhibit cancer cells. It may also lower cholesterol levels, although also lowering HDL ("good") cholesterol.

Quality Concerns and Product Testing

Neither the FDA nor any other federal or state agency routinely tests supplements for quality prior to sale. Therefore, it is important to know that a product contains the ingredients that it claims. Too little and you may not get the expected effect and waste your money. Too much, and you may experience negative effects with certain ingredients.

ConsumerLab.com selected, purchased, and tested 7 CLA supplements. (See the appropriate section in "ConsumerLab.com's Testing Methods and Standards," page 662, for more information.)

Test Findings

Of the seven products tested, one product, Allmax® Nutrition CLA, contained only 75% of its CLA; the six others passed testing. Although Allmax is a Canadian brand, some U.S. retailers also sell it.

Products that were selected for testing and a summary of the results are listed alphabetically in Test Results for CLA (Conjugated Linoleic Acid) Supplements. Also included in the list are other products (indicated with an asterisk) that have met the same criteria through CL's Voluntary Certification Program (see Selection and Testing, page 25, volume 1).

ConsumerTips™ for Buying and Using

Food Sources: CLA is found naturally in milk fat (typically about 5 mg of CLA/gram of fat, but it can range from 2 to 18 mg/gram of fat) and meat fat, (particularly lamb (6 mg/gram), beef (4 mg/gram), and veal (2 mg/gram). Nonfat products will have little CLA. However, increasing the consumption of fatty food sources is obviously not recommended for achieving a high intake of CLA for weight loss.

Supplements: CLA is commonly found along with many other oils in CLA supplements. Make sure that you focus on the "conjugated linoleic acid" content in the Supplement Facts ingredient listings. CLA tends to account for about 75% of the oils in some popular proprietary blends. Various forms or isomers of CLA may perform different functions. The "trans-10, cis-12" form (also known as t10, c12 -octadecadienoic acid) appears to be the form most associated with changes in body composition, but may also have potential side effects (see Concerns and Cautions). This form and another known as cis-9, trans-11 both show preliminary anticancer activity. The effectiveness of a CLA supplement may depend on the proportion of the forms present. However, at this time, most products do not specify the ratio of CLA forms.

Recent studies suggesting improvement in lean body mass used 3 to 4 grams (3,000 to 4,000 mg) a day of CLA. Six grams a day was used to improve insulin levels. If a product includes other oils when showing the amount of CLA on its label, take that information into consideration when calculating the dosage.

Concerns and Cautions

CLA is generally safe in healthy individuals. However, some people report feeling slightly nauseous after taking CLA or have gastrointestinal upset or loose stools. These side effects typically are reduced if CLA is taken with protein (such as milk), and usually decrease after about two weeks of supplementation.

Recent studies have found CLA may worsen blood sugar control in people with diabetes and in obese people without diabetes. Studies also show that CLA may decrease insulin sensitivity, creating a prediabetic state, and lower HDL cholesterol ("good" cholesterol) as well. The form of CLA used in these studies was the trans-10, cis-12 isomer of CLA, the same that has been associated with the slimming effect. Because most commercial CLA products contain a mixture of CLA isomers, it is not known if these products have this same risk. Individuals with diabetes or at risk for it should not use CLA except under physician supervision.

CLA also appears to reduce the fat content of human breast milk. Therefore, it is probably prudent for nursing mothers to avoid taking CLA supplements.

Maximum safe dosages of CLA for young children, pregnant women, or anyone with severe liver or kidney disease have not been determined.

Test Results for CLA (Conjugated Linoleic Acid) Supplements

Product (label info: amount of CLA/unit dosing)‡ Daily amount of CLA (Mf suggested) Manufacturer (Mf) or Distributor (Dist)	Test Results	
	Approved or not approved	Contained labeled amount of CLA
🍁 Allmax® Nutrition CLA (1,000 mg/softgel, 3–6/day) Daily: 3,000–6,000 mg Dist: Allmax Nutrition Inc.	**not** approved	Contained only 75% of labeled amount of CLA**
AST® Sports Science CLA 1000™ (750 mg/softgel, 4–6/day) Daily: 3,000–4,500 mg Dist: AST® Sports Science	approved	✔
Metagenics® Ultra CLA® (500 mg/softgel, 6/day) Daily: 3,000 mg Dist: Metagenics Inc.	approved	✔
Natrol™ Tonalin®, CLA (750 mg/softgel, 3/day) Daily: 2,250 mg Dist: Natrol, Inc.	approved	✔

Product (label info.)	Test Results	
	Approval	**Contained labeled**
Natural Max® Ultra Supertone® CLA 1400 (1,000 mg/softgel, 3/day) Daily: 3,000 mg Mf: Nutraceutical Corp. for NaturalMax	approved	✔
Nature's Sunshine® CLA (750 mg/softgel, 3/day) Daily: 2,250 mg Dist: Nature's Sunshine Products Inc.	approved	✔
Nutrilite® CLA 500 (500 mg/softgel, 6/day)* Daily: 3,000 mg Dist: Access Business Group International LLC	approved	✔
Ultimate Nutrition® Patented CLA Pure™ (750 mg/softgel, 3/day) Daily: 2,250 mg Dist: Ultimate Nutrition, Inc.	approved	✔
Vitamin World® CLA 1000 mg*, NNFA GMP (740 mg/ softgel, 4/day) Daily: 2,960 mg Mf: Vitamin World, Inc.	approved	✔

continued

Product Reviews: Special Ingredients

✔ Check indicates the results met the criteria listed in the column heading.

‡ See also "More Brand Information," page 675.

*Tested through CL's Voluntary Certification Program before, at the time of, or after the initial review.

**After release of this report, the distributor of this product informed ConsumerLab.com that its labeling was incorrect and that newer lots are labeled to explain that the softgel contains 1,000 mg of ingredient of which 77% is CLA. The newly labeled product has not been evaluated by CL but would be consistent (within an acceptable margin of error) with our findings.

🍁 Purchased from a retailer in Canada

Coenzyme Q10

Coenzyme Q10 (CoQ10), also known as ubiquinone, is a naturally occurring antioxidant compound that is used for energy production within cells. It's manufactured in the heart, liver, kidney, and pancreas. The body normally produces sufficient CoQ10, although some medications such as statins may interfere with this process and CoQ10 levels in the body may decline with age and heart disease. Only small amounts of CoQ10 are available from food, mainly beef and chicken. Consequently, dietary supplements are the most common way to increase the body's CoQ10 levels.

Taken orally, coenzyme Q10 may help treat congestive heart failure, a disease in which the heart doesn't adequately maintain circulation. CoQ10's role in cell energy production may be the mechanism by which it assists the heart. CoQ10 may help prevent migraine headaches, reduce the likelihood of more heart problems in some people who've had a first heart attack, and delay the progression of Parkinson's disease. CoQ10 may also be useful in treating other diseases, including muscular dystrophy, AIDS, hypertension, and mitochondrial encephalomyopathies. There is recent evidence that it may increase sperm motility. CoQ10 might help reverse side effects experienced by people who have taken statin drugs to lower high cholesterol. Although sometimes touted for enhancing athletic performance and treating gum disease, these uses haven't been well demonstrated.

More information about the CoQ10's uses and clinical studies is found in the review article in the Encyclopedia on the ConsumerLab .com Web site.

Quality Concerns and Product Testing

No government agency is responsible for routinely testing CoQ10 supplements or other dietary supplements for their contents or quality. Research by ConsumerLab.com in 2000 and 2004 found that not all CoQ10 supplements contained their claimed amounts. Because products on the market are constantly changing, ConsumerLab.com recently evaluated more CoQ10 products to determine whether they contained the amounts of CoQ10 stated on their labels. All non-chewable tablets were also tested to be sure that they would properly disintegrate. (See ConsumerLab.com's Testing Methods and Standards, page 663, for more information.)

Test Findings

All of the products tested were found to contain their labeled amounts of CoQ10. Any product in tablet form (excluding chewables) was also tested to be sure it would break apart properly—the one applicable product passed this testing.

Although all products passed testing, it is important to note that the amount of CoQ10 across products ranged from 15 mg to as much as 400 mg. It is important, therefore, that you determine the proper dose for your intended use rather than rely on a product's suggested serving. (See the ConsumerTips™ for Buying and Using below for dosage information and consult your doctor.) Switching from a low-dose to high-dose product, or vice versa, may affect the efficacy and side effects associated with use of CoQ10.

See "ConsumerLab.com's Testing Methods and Standards," page 663 for more information about testing and criteria. Listed alphabetically in Test Results for CoQ10 Supplements are the test results for 37 CoQ10 supplements. ConsumerLab.com selected 16. Twenty-one others (each indicated with an asterisk) were tested at the request of their manufacturers/distributors through CL's Voluntary Certification Program and are included for having passed testing. Also listed are eight products similar to ones that passed but sold under different brand names.

ConsumerTips™ for Buying and Using

CoQ10 recommended daily dosages vary widely. In this review alone, products provided daily doses ranging from 15 to 400 mg of the substance. When comparing product costs, consider the dosage and number of pills per bottle

Using CoQ10 to treat congestive heart failure should be considered an adjunct to, not a replacement for, other medications; a daily dose of 100 to 200 mg of CoQ10 is generally used, with the dose dependent on the individual's weight. Be aware that improvement in symptoms may take more than one month. Don't suddenly stop taking CoQ10 because symptoms may worsen. Tapering off the supplement is recommended. Similarly, you may want to work up to the full dose over a period of weeks when starting therapy, as some people experience heart pain with full dose therapy.

CoQ10 in a daily dose of 300 mg may help prevent migraine headaches, but doesn't affect the severity or duration of migraines once they begin. It can take up to three months to achieve the full migraine-preventing benefits of CoQ10.

For other diseases, the following daily doses have been used, although optimal dosage levels have not been determined: for Parkinson's disease, 300 to 1,200 mg; for hypertension, 120 to 200 mg; for angina, 150 mg; for reducing the likelihood of future heart problems in people who've had a first heart attack, 120 mg; for HIV/AIDS, 200 mg; for muscular dystrophy, 100 mg; for mitochondrial encephalomyopathies, 150 to 160 mg and sometimes higher; for increasing sperm motility, 200 mg.

CoQ10 might help reverse side effects caused by statins, drugs used to lower high cholesterol. Some of the side effects reportedly reversed with CoQ10 include myalgia (muscle pain), fatigue, dyspnea, memory loss, and peripheral neuropathy. While daily doses for reversing "statin" side effects have not been determined, an average daily dose of 240 mg was reportedly effective in a series of 50 people treated for statin side effects.

Divided dosing (taking two or three equally divided smaller doses instead of one large dose a day) is recommended when the total daily dose exceeds 100 mg.

Research on animals suggests that only a small amount of CoQ10 is actually absorbed. CoQ10, especially the dry dosage form (tablet or capsule), is best absorbed when fats or oils are present in the gastrointestinal tract, so take such supplements with meals. (A softgel isn't considered a dry form.) Products containing CoQ10 dissolved in oil or solubilized in other substances seem to be better absorbed than products containing the dry form.

The CoQ10 found in most supplements is in the oxidized state (ubiquinone), but once in the body it readily goes into the reduced state (ubiquinol). Normally, both forms can be found in your body and the active (reduced) form of CoQ10 is regenerated many times. Currently some products are being sold as ubiquinol, but not much research has been done to show that it gets into your body as well as CoQ10 (as ubiquinone).

Naturally formed CoQ10 is 100% in the trans isomer form, while the synthetically formed material is approximately 50% in the trans form and 50% in the cis form. Some synthetic CoQ10 was found in the market a few years ago, but now the CoQ10 found in the marketplace is made by a fermentation process. Since the fermentation process using bacteria or yeast is much cheaper than chemical synthesis and provides 100% natural (trans) CoQ10, it is unlikely that a product today will contain synthetic CoQ10.

Concerns and Cautions

CoQ10 is generally safe when taken by adults in appropriate amounts, but its safety has not been evaluated for pregnant or breast-feeding women. CoQ10 has been used safely in children, under medical supervision, in doses up to 10 mg/kg/day for up to nine months.

Individuals with diabetes and those taking blood thinners are strongly advised to consult a physician before taking this supplement, because of potential drug interactions.

Certain medications, including some cholesterol-lowering statin drugs, beta-blockers, antidepressants, and antipsychotics may decrease the body's natural production of CoQ10; therefore, the CoQ10 dosage for individuals taking any of these drugs might be higher than generally recommended.

Test Results for CoQ10 Supplements

Product (label info: amount of elemental CoQ10 per unit, dose)‡ Manufacturer (Mf) or Distributor (Dist)	Test Results	
	Approved or not approved	Contained claimed amount of CoQ10
AllergyResearchGroup® Coenzyme Q10, 50 mg with Vitamin C, Hypoallergenic (50 mg per capsule, 2–6/day) Daily: 100–300 mg Dist: Allergy Research Group®	approved	✔
Berkley & Jensen® CoQ10 100 mg (100 mg per softgel, 1/day) Daily: 100 mg Dist: BJWC	approved	✔
Bioenhanced DOUBLE STRENGTH LiQ-10™ Syrup, Orange Pineapple Flavor, Formulated with Li-Q-Sorb™ Liposomal CoQ10 (100 mg per teaspoon [5 mL], 1–3 tsp/day)* Daily: 100–300 mg Mf: Tishcon Corp.	approved	✔

continued

471

Product Reviews: Special Ingredients

Product (label info.)	Test Results	
	Approval	Contained claimed
Bluebonnet CoQ10 100 mg Softgels (100 mg per softgel, 1/day) Daily: 100 mg Dist: Bluebonnet Nutrition Corporation	approved	✔
Carlson® CO-Q10 50 mg (50 mg per softgel, 1/day)* Daily: 50 mg Dist: Carlson Division of J.R. Carlson Laboratories, Inc.	approved	✔
Carni Q-Gel® FORTE Coenzyme Q-10 30 mg, + L-Carnitine Fumarate 440 mg, Bio-Solv® (30 mg per softsule, 1–2/day)* Daily: 30–60 mg Mf: Gel-Tec, Division of Tishcon Corp.	approved	✔
Doctor's BEST® High Absorption CoQ10 100 mg, with BIOPERINIE® (100 mg per capsule, 1/day) Daily: 100 mg Dist: Doctor's Best, Inc.	approved	✔

Product (label info.)	Test Results	
	Approval	**Contained claimed**
Gary Null's Super Coenzyme Q10 100 mg (100 mg per tablet, 1–2/day) Daily: 100–200 mg Dist: Gary Null & Associates	approved	✔
GNC Preventive Nutrition® CoQ-10 100 mg (100 mg per capsule, 1/day)* Daily: 100 mg Dist: General Nutrition Corporation	approved	✔
Healthy Origins® 100% Natural (trans-isomer) CoQ10 Gels 100 mg, Kaneka Q10 The Natural One™ (100 mg per softgel capsule, 1–2/day) Daily: 100–200 mg Dist: Healthy Origins	approved	✔
Inno-Vite CoQ-10 M.R.B Maximum Relative Bioavailability Q-Gel® Forte 30 mg (30 mg per softsule, 1/day) Daily: 30 mg Dist: INNO-VITE Inc.	approved	✔

continued

Product Reviews: Special Ingredients

Product (label info.)	Test Results	
	Approval	Contained claimed
Longs® Wellness, Coenzyme Q10 50 mg (50 mg per softgel, 1–3/ day) Daily: 50–150 mg Dist: Longs Drugs	approved	✔
Nature Made® CoQ10 (200 mg CoQ10/softgel 1/day) Daily: 200 mg Dist: Nature Made Nutritional Products	approved	✔
Nature's Bounty ® Q-SORB™ Co Q-10 75 mg (75 mg per softgel, 2/day)* Daily: 150 mg Mf: Nature's Bounty, Inc.	approved	✔
Nature's Bounty® Q-SORB™ Co Q-10 120 mg (120 mg per softgel, 1/day)* Daily: 120 mg Mf: Nature's Bounty, Inc.	approved	✔

Product (label info.)	Test Results	
	Approval	Contained claimed
PhytoPharmica Natural Medicines® CoQ10 50 mg (50 mg per softgel capsule, 3/day) Daily: 150 mg Dist: PhytoPharmica, Div. of Integrative Therapeutics, Inc.	approved	✔
Pro Health™ Coenzyme Q10; Selenium and E in an Enhanced Absorption Base; 50 mg (50 mg per softgel, 1–2/day) Daily: 50–100 mg Dist: Pro Health, Inc.	approved	✔
Puritan's Pride® Q-Sorb™ Co Q-10 200 mg (200 mg per softgel, 1/day)* Daily: 200 mg Mf: Puritan's Pride, Inc.	approved	✔
Puritan's Pride® Q-Sorb™ Co Q-10 30 mg (30 mg per softgel, 3/day)* Daily: 90 mg Dist: Puritan's Pride, Inc.	approved	✔

continued

Product Reviews: Special Ingredients

Product (label info.)	Test Results	
	Approval	**Contained claimed**
Q-Gel® Bio Solv® Coenzyme Q10 15 mg (15 mg per softsule, 1–3/day)* Daily: 15–45 mg Mf: Gel-Tec Division of Tishcon Corp.	approved	✔
Q-Gel® FORTE Bio Solv® Coenzyme Q10 30 mg (30 mg per softsule, 1–3/day)* Daily: 30–90 mg Mf: Gel-Tec Division of Tishcon Corp.	approved	✔
Q-Gel® MEGA 100 Bio Solv® Coenzyme Q10 100 mg (100 mg per softsule, 1/day)* Daily: 100 mg Mf: Gel-Tec Division of Tishcon Corp.	approved	✔
Q-Gel® Ultra Bio Solv® Coenzyme Q10 60 mg +150 IU Vitamin E, USP (60 mg per softsule, 1–3/day)* Daily: 60–180 mg Mf: Gel-Tec Division of Tishcon Corp.	approved	✔

Product (label info.)	Test Results	
	Approval	Contained claimed
Rite Aid Coenzyme Q-10, Natural, 30 mg (30 mg per softgel, 1/day) Daily: 30 mg Dist: Rite Aid Corporation	approved	✔
Shaklee® CoenzymeQ10, Resveratrol, & More; CoQHEART® (30 mg per softgel, 1/day) Daily: 30 mg Dist: Shaklee Corporation	approved	✔
Spring Valley® Q-Sorb™ CoQ-10 150 mg (150 mg per softgel, 1/day)* Daily: 150 mg Mf: Nature's Bounty, Inc.	approved	✔
SUGAR FREE Chew Q® 100 mg Bioenhanced Coenzyme Q10 (100 mg per chewtab, 1/day)* Daily: 100 mg Mf: Tishcon Corp.	approved	✔
SUGAR FREE Chew Q® 30 mg Vegetarian Bioenhanced Coenzyme Q10 (30 mg per chewtab, 1/day)* Daily: 30 mg Mf: Tishcon Corp.	approved	✔

continued

Product (label info.)	Test Results	
	Approval	Contained claimed
Sugar-Free, From the Makers of Q-Gel®, Clinically Tested Liquid Q LiQsorb™ Drops, Enhanced absorption (15 mg per 6 drops [0.167 mL], 6 drops/day)* Daily: 15 mg Mf: Tishcon Corp.	approved	✔
Sundown® Easy to Swallow Q-Sorb™ CoQ10 100 mg (100 mg per softgel, 1/day)* Daily: 100 mg Mf: Sundown, Inc.	approved	✔
Sundown® Easy to Swallow Q-Sorb™ CoQ10 50 mg (50 mg per softgel, 2/day)* Daily: 100 mg Mf: Sundown, Inc.	approved	✔
Trace Minerals Research Liqumins™ Fast-Absorbing Liquid Co-Q10, Natural Orange Cream Flavor (50 mg per teaspoon [5 mL], 1 tsp/day) Daily: 50 mg Dist: Trace Minerals Research	approved	✔

Product (label info.)	Test Results	
	Approval	Contained claimed
USANA® Optimizers CoQuinone® 30 (30 mg per softgel, 1–2/day) Daily: 30–60 mg Mf: USANA Health Sciences, Inc.	approved	✔
Vitamin World® Naturally Inspired™ Q-Sorb™ Coenzyme Q-10 50 mg (50 mg per softgel, 2–3/day)* Daily: 100–150 mg Mf: Vitamin World, Inc.	approved	✔
Vitamin World® Naturally Inspired™ Super Potency Coenzyme Q-10 400 mg (400 mg per softgel, 1/day)* Daily: 400 mg Mf: Vitamin World, Inc.	approved	✔
Vitanica® Natural CoQ10 100 mg CoQ10 Extra (100 mg per capsule, 1/day) Daily: 100 mg Dist: Vitanica	approved	✔

continued

Product Reviews: Special Ingredients

Product (label info.)	Test Results	
	Approval	**Contained claimed**
Vitasmart® Coenzyme Q-10 100 mg (100 mg per softgel, 1/day) Daily: 100 mg Dist: Kmart Corporation	approved	✔

Similar to Approved Products**

Nature's Bounty® Q-SORB™ Co Q-10 30 mg Heart Healthy (30 mg per softgel, 3/day)*

Mf: Nature's Bounty, Inc.

Nature's Bounty® Q-SORB™ Co Q-10 50 mg Heart Healthy (50 mg per softgel, 2–3/day)*

Mf: Nature's Bounty, Inc.

Nature's Bounty® Q-SORB™ Heart Healthy Co Q-10 200 mg (200 mg per softgel, 1/day)*

Mf: Nature's Bounty, Inc.

Puritan's Pride Cardio Q10® Super Potency Q-Sorb™ Coenzyme Q-10 400 mg (400 mg per softgel, 1/day)*

Mf: Puritan's Pride, Inc.

Puritan's Pride Q-Sorb™ COENZYME Q-10 50 mg (50 mg per softgel, 2–3/day)*

Mf: Puritan's Pride, Inc.

Vitamin World Naturally Inspired® Q-Sorb™ Coenzyme Q-10 120 mg (120 mg per softgel, 1/day)*

Mf: Vitamin World, Inc.

Product (label info.)	Test Results	
	Approval	**Contained claimed**
Vitamin World® Naturally Inspired® Q-Sorb™ Coenzyme Q-10 75 mg (75 mg per softgel, 2/day)* Mf: Vitamin World, Inc.		
Vitamin World® Naturally Inspired™ Q-SORB™Q-10 200 mg (200 mg per softgel, 1/day)* Mf: Vitamin World, Inc.		

*Tested through CL's Voluntary Certification Program prior to, at time of, or after initial posting of this Product Review.

**Product identical in formulation and manufacture to a product that has passed testing but sold under a different brand. For more information on CL's Multi-Label Testing Program see Selection and Testing section, page 25, volume 1.

‡ See also "More Brand Information," page 675.

✔ Check indicates the results met the criteria listed in the column heading.

DHEA

Dehydroepiandrosterone (DHEA) is a hormone produced in the body by the adrenal glands. DHEA in dietary supplements is synthetic, manufactured from plant chemicals found in soybeans and wild yams. You cannot, however, get DHEA directly from eating soy or yams. Other names for DHEA are prasterone and DHEA sulfate. A pharmaceutical-grade preparation trademarked Prestara™ (formerly known as Aslera™ or GL701) has been developed and is in clinical trials for potential use on a prescription basis. Be aware that 7-keto DHEA (used in some weight-loss supplements and reviewed separately by ConsumerLab.com) is not the same as DHEA.

Anti-Aging: The body uses DHEA to produce other steroidal hormones, such as estrogen and testosterone, after first converting it into androstenedione. Levels of DHEA peak in a person's twenties, and then begin to decline. On this basis, DHEA supplements have been touted as a kind of "fountain of youth," said to reverse the effects of aging.

DHEA, however, is not a general anti-aging solution. In more than ten double-blind studies enrolling thousands of seniors, DHEA supplementation has failed to improve general well-being, muscle mass, or mental function. On the other hand, there is weak evidence that DHEA, in women over age 70, might help improve sexual dysfunction and help prevent or treat osteoporosis. In elderly men and women, DHEA may also increase skin thickness and hydration as well as decrease facial skin pigmentation. DHEA may also improve erectile dysfunction in men who have low DHEA levels (see "Sexual-Enhancement Supplements"). Very weak evidence hints that when given to seniors, DHEA might enhance the immune response to vaccines.

SLE: The best evidence for benefit with DHEA involves people with the autoimmune disease lupus (systemic lupus erythematosus or SLE). SLE is estimated to affect up to 1.5 million Americans. The vast majority of those afflicted with SLE are women. According to several studies, DHEA may permit a reduction of the normal dose of corticosteroid medication. Initial research suggested that it might also offset side effects of corticosteroid therapy such as accelerated osteoporosis, but a 6-month study showed no statistical benefit over placebo.

Growing evidence suggests that DHEA might also be helpful for depression. The largest study involved 145 people with HIV/AIDS as well as mild depression. Over a period of eight weeks, use of DHEA at a dose of up to 400 mg daily significantly improved symptoms as compared to placebo. A much smaller study found it possibly helpful for midlife onset of major and minor depression.

According to two studies by a single research group, DHEA may enhance the effectiveness and reduce the side effects of medications used for treatment of schizophrenia.

According to some, but not all, studies of women with adrenal failure, DHEA may help improve mood and bone density when used in conjunction with standard hormone replacement therapy. DHEA has also shown promise as an additional hormonal treatment in pituitary failure.

There is preliminary evidence that DHEA might also be helpful in chronic fatigue syndrome. Most studies of DHEA in athletic performance and as a weight-loss aid have not shown a benefit— although DHEA remains banned from use in Olympic athletes and in the National Basketball Association. 7-keto DHEA (a metabolite of DHEA that cannot be converted into estrogen or testosterone) may have application in weight loss, although the evidence is preliminary (see "Weight-Loss Supplements," page 202, volume 1).

There is evidence that DHEA could potentially contribute to plaque formation in arteries. See ConsumerTips™ for Buying and Using, page 484.

Quality Concerns and Product Testing

During the manufacture of DHEA, other steroid-like compounds may be produced, such as androstenedione (andro), contaminating the DHEA. In addition, there have been reports of supplements (particularly those marketed for athletic enhancement) having undeclared steroid-like compounds. Neither the FDA nor any other federal or state agency routinely tests supplements for quality prior to sale. Consequently, ConsumerLab.com tested DHEA products to determine if they met label claims for amounts of DHEA and to evaluate their purity. Tablets and caplets were also tested to be sure that they could disintegrate properly for absorption (See "ConsumerLab.com's Testing Methods and Standards," page 664, for more information.)

Test Results

All of the products, except one, contained their labeled amounts of DHEA, which ranged from 25 mg to 100 mg per suggested daily serving. Only Natural 99% Pure DHEA, however, contained a much greater amount of DHEA than claimed on its label. Our testing found 21.5 mg of DHEA instead of the 10 mg per capsule—215% of the labeled amount stated on the label.

Tablets were tested for their ability to properly break apart (disintegrate) and all passed this testing. All products also passed testing limits for contamination with androstenedione (an FDA controlled substance) and related anabolic compounds.

Test Findings

Listed alphabetically in the table Test Results for DHEA Supplements are the findings for 11 DHEA products. ConsumerLab.com selected 9. Two others (each indicated with an asterisk) were tested at the request of their manufacturers/distributors through CL's Voluntary Certification Program and are included for having passed testing. Also listed are three products similar to ones that passed but sold under different brand names.

ConsumerTips™ for Buying and Using

The labeled amount of DHEA in products may vary considerably. Among products evaluated in this review, labeled amounts ranged from 10 mg to 100 mg per pill. Purchase a product that will conveniently provide the appropriate dose for the intended use. Do not confuse 7-Keto DHEA with DHEA, as they are different compounds and have different biologic activities.

Some products contain "bioperine," a purported bioavailability-enhancing phytonutrient from *Piper nigrum* fruit (black pepper). The manufacturer of bioperine claims that it increases the absorption of certain supplement ingredients. However, ConsumerLab.com was not able to find research supporting its ability to specifically increase DHEA absorption.

Although now seldom found, some products may claim to contain bovine (cow) adrenal gland concentrate. Due to concerns relating to mad cow disease (bovine spongiform encephalopathy) and variant Creutzfeldt-Jakob disease in humans, you should avoid products made from cow glands, unless you can be certain that animal source was free of infection, which is difficult to ascertain.

Dosage: The following are the dosages used to treat several conditions:

For lupus (SLE), 200 mg daily as an adjunct to conventional therapy. Higher doses have also been used. For depression, 100–450 mg daily, along with standard therapy; for adrenal insufficiency 50 mg daily, along with standard therapy; for pituitary insufficiency, 50 mg daily, along with standard therapy; for sexual dysfunction, 50 mg daily; to prevent osteoporosis, 25 to 50 mg daily; to augment effectiveness of medications for schizophrenia, 100 mg daily.

A cream containing 10% DHEA has been used vaginally in a dose of 3 to 5 grams daily in postmenopausal women in hopes that it can treat vaginal atrophy and increase bone density.

Concerns and Cautions

At doses up to 200 mg daily, DHEA appears to be generally safe, at least in the short term (up to one year). However, you should be aware of the following potential side effects and drug interactions.

Some (but not all) studies have found that DHEA, even at the low dose of 25 mg per day, may decrease levels of HDL (good) cholesterol. And a report in 2003 suggested that DHEA might increase the formation of certain cells (foam cells) known to contribute to plaque formation in blood vessels, potentially raising a person's risk of heart disease.

DHEA may increase testosterone levels in women, leading to acne, hair loss, voice deepening, and changes in menstrual pattern in some women. Rare cases of liver dysfunction, abdominal pain, hypertension, insomnia, and arrhythmia have also been reported. There have been rare cases of mania reported, although sometimes not occurring until after months of use.

Women with hormone-sensitive diseases such as breast cancer should use DHEA with caution, as it can be converted into estrogen. There is also concern that long term and/or high-dose use might increase the risk of breast cancer. Associations have also been found between higher DHEA levels and both prostate cancer and ovarian cancer.

DHEA might, in theory, increase blood levels of any of the many hundreds of medications that are metabolized by cytochrome P450 3A.

DHEA might increase insulin resistance or, conversely, insulin sensitivity. Blood glucose should be monitored by diabetics using DHEA.

Safety in pregnant or nursing women or people with severe liver or kidney disease has not been established.

Use of DHEA is banned by the International Olympic Committee and the National Basketball Association because of its potential use as a performance enhancer and its potential conversion into other steroid-like compounds.

Test Results for DHEA Supplements

Product (label info: amount of DHEA per unit, dose)‡ Manufacturer (Mf) or Distributor (Dist)	Test Results		
	Approved or not approved	Contained claimed amount of DHEA found in daily dose	Broke apart properly
AST Sports Science DHEA 100™ Dehydroepiandrosterone (100 mg DHEA per capsule, 1/day) Dist: AST® Sports Science	approved	✔	N/A
Doctor's Trust® Vitamins DHEA 25 mg (25 mg DHEA per capsule, 1/day) Dist: Doctor's Trust® Vitamins	approved	✔	N/A
Natrol™ DHEA 25 mg, HPLC Verified, Tested for Purity (25 mg DHEA per tablet, 1/day) Mf: NATROL, Inc	approved	✔	✔
Nature's Bounty® DHEA 25 mg (25 mg DHEA per tablet, 1/day)* Mf: Nature's Bounty	approved	✔	✔

continued

Product (label info.)	Test Results		
	Approval	Contained claimed	Broke apart properly
Only Natural 99% Pure DHEA (Dehydro-epiandrosterone) 10 mg (10 mg DHEA per capsule, 1/day) Dist: Only Natural, Inc.	**not** approved	Contained 215% of claimed amount of DHEA (21.5 mg per capsule)	N/A
PHD DHEA Plus (50 mg DHEA per enteric coated tablet, 1/day) Dist: Wellness International Network, Ltd	approved	✔	N/A
PhysioLogics® DHEA, Doctor Recommended, Dehydroepiandrosterone 25 mg (25 mg DHEA per capsule, 1/day) Mf: Physiologics	approved	✔	N/A
Puritan's Pride® DHEA 50 mg Dehydroepian-drosterone (50 mg DHEA per tablet, 1/day)* Mf: Puritan's Pride	approved	✔	✔
Smart Basics DHEA, 25 mg (25 mg DHEA per capsule, 1/day) Dist: Vitacost.com	approved	✔	N/A
Solaray® DHEA with MexiYam®, 25 mg DHEA, 370 mg MexiYam® Root (25 mg DHEA per capsule, 1/day) Mf: Nutraceutical Corp.	approved	✔	N/A

Product (label info.)	Test Results		
	Approval	Contained claimed	Broke apart properly
TriMedica® DHEA 50 mg (50 mg DHEA per capsule, 1/day) Dist: TriMedica™, Inc.	approved	✔	N/A

Similar to Approved Products**

Puritan's Pride® DHEA 25 mg Dehydroepiandrosterone (25 mg DHEA per tablet, 1/day)*

Mf: Puritan's Pride

Vitamin World® Naturally Inspired™ DHEA 25 mg Dehydroepiandrosterone (25 mg DHEA per tablet, 1/day)*

Dist: Vitamin World

Vitamin World® Naturally Inspired™ DHEA 50 mg Dehydroepiandrosterone, Vegetarian Formula (50 mg DHEA per tablet, 1/day)*

Dist: Vitamin World

‡ See also "More Brand Information," page 675.

*Tested through CL's Voluntary Certification Program prior to, at time of, or after initial posting of this Product Review.

**Product identical in formulation and manufacture to a product that has passed testing but sold under a different brand. For more information on CL's Multi-Label Testing Program, see Selection and Testing section, page 25, volume 1.

✔ Check indicates the results met the criteria listed in the column heading.

Melatonin Supplements

Melatonin (N-acetyl-5-methoxytryptamine), synthesized from the amino acid tryptophan, is a hormone produced by the pineal gland in the brain. Some foods contain extremely tiny amounts of melatonin. The melatonin in dietary supplements is generally manufactured synthetically or extracted from plants; however, it is chemically identical to the melatonin in your body.

Melatonin is known to play a role in regulating the body's natural wake-sleep cycle (circadian rhythm), triggering sleep. Levels of melatonin increase as exposure to light decreases, and decrease as light exposure increases. On this basis, melatonin has been proposed as a treatment for people whose natural sleep cycles have been disturbed. Inconsistent evidence suggests that it may aid sleep in jet travelers who have crossed several time zones. However, study results have not been impressive in treatment of sleep disorders related to shift work, general insomnia for adults, or insomnia in seniors. Nevertheless, some benefit has been seen in specific conditions such as sleep disorders in blind individuals and in children with developmental disabilities, such as autism, delayed sleep phase syndrome (DSPS, a condition in which people cannot fall asleep till early morning), and delayed weekend sleep pattern (difficulty falling asleep Sunday night after staying up late Friday and Saturday night).

Melatonin has also shown promise in treatment of children with chronic sleep problems, for people withdrawing from sleep-aid medications, and for improving sleep in people with diabetes, schizophrenia, Alzheimer's, or Parkinson's, or who are hospitalized. Valerian is another supplement used for insomnia and sometimes included in melatonin supplements (see "Valerian," page 297, volume 1).

Other potential uses for melatonin include reducing preoperative anxiety, symptoms of tardive dyskinesia (a potential long-term side effect of antipsychotic medications), nicotine withdrawal symptoms, irritable bowel syndrome, and cluster headaches. Additionally, preliminary evidence suggests that melatonin may also be useful as an adjunct to conventional therapy in treating some forms of cancer, reducing side effects or enhancing drug efficacy. Melatonin also has antioxidant properties. According to some reports, melatonin levels drop with age and on this basis melatonin has been recommended as an "anti-aging" supplement. However, recent evidence suggests that melatonin levels do not, in fact, alter with age.

Quality Concerns and Product Testing

Neither the FDA nor any other federal or state agency routinely tests supplements for quality prior to sale.

ConsumerLab.com tested melatonin products to determine if they met label claims and did not contain unacceptable levels of lead, a potential contaminant. Standard tablets were also tested to be sure that they could disintegrate, or break apart properly (see the appropriate section in "ConsumerLab.com's Testing Methods and Standards," page 665, for more information).

Test Findings

Among the supplements that ConsumerLab.com selected for testing, all contained their claimed amounts of melatonin, although these amounts ranged from 200 mcg to 3,000 mcg (1,000 mcg = 1 mg). All standard tablets properly broke apart. In addition, all products passed testing for lead contamination. (See the appropriate section in "ConsumerLab.com's Testing Methods and Standards," page 665.)

The 14 products that were selected for testing and a summary of the results are listed alphabetically in Test Results for Melatonin Supplements. Also included in the list are 6 other products (indicated with an asterisk) that have met the same criteria through CL's Voluntary Certification Program (see Selection and Testing, page 25, volume 1). Also listed are 10 products that are the same as ones that passed but are sold under different brand names.

ConsumerTips™ for Buying and Using

Most melatonin supplements are synthetically manufactured but chemically identical to the melatonin produced in the body. Supplements are required to list their source of melatonin if made directly from plant or animal sources. If the source is not given, it is assumed to be synthetic. Consequently, supplements that say "vegetarian" or "nonanimal" melatonin but don't list the specific source are likely to be synthetic melatonin. Melatonin extracted from animal glands carries potential infection with the prion that causes mad cow disease and variant Creutzfeldt-Jakob disease in humans. Transmission of this disease from supplements, however, has not been documented.

The full chemical name for melatonin is "N-acetyl-5-methoxytryptamine." Some products state "5-methoxy-tryptamine," and others just state "melatonin"—all three are synonymous.

The labeled amount of melatonin in products can range significantly from just a couple of hundred micrograms (mcg) to three thousand micrograms a pill. Purchase a product that will conveniently provide the appropriate dose for the intended use.

Melatonin is available in quick-release form, regular tablets, capsules, and special time-release forms that extend its release over several hours (also referred to as extended-release or controlled-release). Quick-release aids the ability to fall asleep, and time-release may be more helpful in staying asleep. Quick-release products generally cost $.05 to $.10 a day, and time-release products cost a bit more—$.10 to $.25 a day.

Other ingredients in melatonin products may include herbs of a calming reputation, such as valerian, which may promote sleep (see "Valerian," page 297, volume 1). Vitamin B-6 is added to some products, presumably because of its role in the synthesis of serotonin, a melatonin precursor. However, the value of vitamin B-6 in such products seems unclear.

Dosage: These are some of the commonly used dosages for melatonin.

To aid in falling asleep, typically 2 to 3 mg (1 mg = 1,000 mcg) melatonin taken one half-hour to one hour before bedtime (although recommendations vary from 0.5 to 5 mg). This dose should be taken for four days following travel to counter insomnia from a long flight. A sustained release form in a dosage of 3 mg may also be combined with an immediate release form at a dosage of 2–3 mg. Dosages less than 2 mg may not be effective. To treat insomnia in children with developmental disorders, 5 mg at 8 PM daily (this was the timing used in a clinical trial that showed some benefit).

To prevent cluster headache, 10 mg before bedtime daily.

As an adjunct in cancer chemotherapy, 10 to 50 mg daily has been used prior to and during therapy.

To reduce tardive dyskinesia, 10 mg daily of time-release form.

For irritable bowel syndrome, 3 mg at bedtime daily.

For delayed weekend sleep pattern, 6 mg 5½ hours before the desired Sunday bedtime.

Concerns and Cautions

Although melatonin has been found to be generally safe, at least in short-term uses, it is a hormone and, like any hormone, could potentially have wide-ranging effects in the body such as the following.

Testosterone and estrogen metabolism may be affected, impairing sperm function in men. In very high doses (over 75 mg daily), melatonin might prevent ovulation in women.

Drowsiness and impaired mental alertness and balance may occur for about six hours after use, although there does not appear to be a "hangover" effect the following day. Nevertheless, you should not drive or operate heavy machinery for several hours after use. People who use sedating drugs should use melatonin only under the supervision of a physician.

Insulin action may be impaired in nondiabetics, although one study found no problem in people with diabetes.

Blood pressure may increase in people taking antihypertensive medications.

There is weak theoretical evidence that melatonin might increase symptoms of nighttime asthma, though more direct research failed to find any problem. It is also theorized, but not proven, that people with autoimmune diseases such as lupus or rheumatoid arthritis should not take melatonin supplements and that melatonin could cause potential problems in people with depression or schizophrenia.

Melatonin's safety in young children, pregnant or nursing women, or people with severe liver or kidney disease has not been established.

Test Results for Melatonin Supplements

Product (label info: amount of melatonin/ unit, dosing)‡ Daily†: amount of Mf suggested melatonin Manufacturer (Mf) or Distributor (Dist)	Test Results		
	Approved or not approved	Contained labeled amount of melatonin	Accept-able level of lead
BioChem® Melatonin (3,000 mcg/rapid release tablet,1/day) Daily: 3,000 mcg Dist: Country Life	approved	✔	✔
Designs for Health Melatonin (3,000 mcg/tablet, 1/day) Daily: 3,000 mcg Mf: Designs for Health, Inc.	approved	✔	✔
Health Yourself® Controlled-Release Melatonin (2,000 mcg/tablet, 1/day) Daily: 2,000 mcg Mf: HVL, Inc.	approved	✔	✔
Innovative Natural Products® Liquid Melatonin (3,000 mcg/mL of liquid, 1/day) Daily: 3,000 mcg Dist: Innovative Natural Products	approved	✔	✔

Product (label info.)	Test Results		
	Approval	Contained labeled	Accept-able level
Lorna Vanderhaeghe SleepSense™, 3,000–9,000 mcg (3,000 mcg/sublingual tablet, 1–3/day) Dist: Preferred Nutrition	approved	✔	✔
Melatonin Sleep™ Dietary Supplement (500 mcg/ chewable tablet, 1/day) Daily: 500 mcg Dist: Northwest Natural Products Inc.	approved	✔	✔
Natural Balance® Herbal Slumber (1,000 mcg/ capsule, 2/day) Daily: 2,000 mcg Dist: Natural Balance	approved	✔	✔
Nature Made® Melatonin 3 mg (3,000 mcg/tablet, 1/day)* Daily: 3,000 mcg Dist: Nature Made	approved	✔	✔
Nature's Bounty® Melatonin 3 mg (3,000 mcg/tablet, 1/day)* Daily: 3,000 mcg Mf: Nature's Bounty, Inc.	approved	✔	✔

continued

Product (label info.)	Test Results		
	Approval	**Contained labeled**	**Accept-able level**
Now® Melatonin 3 mg, 3,000 mcg (3,000 mcg/capsule, 1/day) Mf: Now Foods	approved	✔	✔
Pharmanex® NightTime Formula with Theanine (500 mcg/capsule, 2/day)* Daily: 1,000 mcg Dist: Pharmanex, LLC	approved; also approved for valerian	✔	✔
Puritan's Pride® Melatonin (200 mcg/tablet, 1/day)* Daily: 200 mcg Dist: Puritan's Pride Inc.	approved	✔	✔
❦ Quest Melatonin (3,000 mcg/tablet, 1–3/day) Daily: 3,000–9,000 mcg Mf: Quest Vitamins	approved	✔	✔
Sundown® Melatonin (300 mcg/tablet, 2/day)* Daily: 600 mcg Mf: Sundown, Inc.	approved	✔	✔
Sunsource® Melatonex® (3,000 mcg/time-release tablet, 1/day) Daily: 3,000 mcg Dist: Chattem, Inc.	approved	✔	✔

Product (label info.)	Test Results		
	Approval	Contained labeled	Accept-able level
Trader Darwin's® Chewable Peppermint Flavored Melatonin (500 mcg/ chewable tablet, 1/day) Daily: 500 mcg Dist: Trader Joe's	approved	✔	✔
TriMedica® Deep Dreams™ (3,000 mcg/tablet [combination of "immediate" and "postponed" availability], 1/day) Daily: 3,000 mcg Dist: Trimedica, Inc.	approved	✔	✔
Twinlab® Melatonin Caps (3,000 mcg/capsule, 1/day) Daily: 3,000 mcg Mf: Ideasphere Inc.	approved	✔	✔
Unicity Melatonin (2,500 mcg/sublingual tablet, 1/day) Daily: 2,500 mcg Dist: UniCity	approved	✔	✔
Vitamin World® Melatonin 1 mg (1,000 mcg/tablet, 1/day)* Daily: 1,000 mcg Dist: Vitamin World, Inc.	approved	✔	✔

continued

Product (label info.)	Test Results		
	Approval	Contained labeled	Accept-able level
Similar to Approved Products:**			
Good 'N Natural® Melatonin 1 mg (1,000 mcg/tablet, 1/day) Mf: Good 'N Natural Manufacturing Corp.			
Good 'N Natural® Melatonin 3 mg (3,000 mcg/tablet, 1/day) Mf: Good 'N Natural Manufacturing Corp.			
Nature's Bounty® Melatonin 200 mcg (200 mcg/tablet, 1/day) Mf: Nature's Bounty, Inc.			
Nature's Bounty® Melatonin 1 mg (1,000 mcg/tablet, 1/day) Mf: Nature's Bounty, Inc.			
PhysioLogics® Melatonin 1 mg, Doctor Recommended (1,000 mcg/tablet, 1/day) Mf: PhysioLogics			
Puritan's Pride® Melatonin 1 mg (1,000 mcg/tablet, 1/day) Mf: Puritan's Pride			
Puritan's Pride® Melatonin 3 mg (3,000 mcg/tablet, 1/day) Mf: Puritan's Pride			
Sundown® Melatonin 3 mg (3,000 mcg/tablet, 1/day) Mf: Sundown, Inc.			
Vitamin World® Melatonin 200 mcg (200 mcg/tablet, 1/day) Dist: Vitamin World, Inc.			

Product (label info.)	Test Results		
	Approval	Contained labeled	Accept-able level

Vitamin World® Melatonin 3 mg, Vegetarian Formula (3,000 mcg/tablet, 1/day)

Dist: Vitamin World, Inc.

---

†—1,000 mcg = 1 mg

* Tested through CL's Voluntary Certification Program before, at the time of, or after the initial review.

N/A—Not applicable: Disintegration test applies only to tablets and caplets. Not applicable to chewable products, powders, capsules, liquid, and time-release forms.

✔ Check indicates the results met the criteria listed in the column heading.

‡ See also "More Brand Information," page 675.

🍁 Purchased from a retailer in Canada.

** Product identical in formulation and manufacture to a product that has passed testing but sold under a different brand.

Omega-3 Fatty Acids (EPA and DHA) from Fish Oils

EPA (eicosapentaenoic acid) and DHA (docosahexaenoic acid) are the two principal fatty acids found in fish. They belong to a family of essential nutrients known as omega-3 fatty acids. DHA can also be obtained from other marine sources, such as algae (algal oil). EPA and DHA are polyunsaturated fats ("good" fats, as opposed to saturated fats, which are thought to increase the risk of heart disease). The body can manufacture both EPA and DHA from another essential fatty acid, alpha-linolenic acid (ALA)—found in flaxseed oil, canola oil, soy oil, and walnut oil—but only to a limited extent. (For more information see "Omega-3 and -6 Fatty Acids from Seed Oils as Sources of ALA and GLA," page 271, volume 1.) Omega-3 fatty acids have been reported as helpful in treating numerous conditions.

Cardiovascular Disease: Omega-3 fatty acids have been most widely studied regarding their effects on cardiovascular health. Although results of studies have been somewhat inconsistent, it appears on balance that increased consumption of fish oil may help slow the progression of atherosclerosis and, thereby, prevent heart attacks and reduce risk of sudden death due to cardiac arrythmias. Omega-3 fatty acids have a number of heart-healthy effects, including reducing triglyceride levels, raising levels of HDL ("good") cholesterol and possibly "thinning" the blood, reducing levels of homocysteine, and reducing blood pressure. Fish oils also appear to enhance the effectiveness of statin drugs used to improve cholesterol profile. The U.S. Food and Drug Administration (FDA) permits supplements containing omega-3 fatty acids to make the following statement: "The scientific evidence about whether omega-3 fatty acids may reduce the risk of coronary heart disease is suggestive, but not conclusive." A similar claim was approved in September 2004 for foods with fish oils.

Arthritis and Other Inflammatory Diseases: Increased intake of the omega-3 fatty acids in fish oil alter the body's production of substances known as prostaglandins, and consequently reduce some forms of inflammation. On the basis of this, EPA and DHA have been tried in the treatment of symptoms of rheumatoid arthritis with considerable success (especially in early stages of the disease). Unlike disease-modifying drugs, however, fish oil probably doesn't slow the progression of the disease.

The anti-inflammatory effects of EPA and DHA have also caused researchers to investigate possible benefits of fish oil for the treatment of menstrual cramps, inflammatory bowel disease (ulcerative colitis and Crohn's disease), lupus, and IgA nephropathy. For each of these conditions, at least one double-blind study has found positive results.

Psychiatric and Mental Disorders: For reasons that are less clear, omega-3s seem to help depression, bipolar disorder, and schizophrenia, according to a limited number of double-blind trials. Fish oil has also been proposed for attention deficit disorder, borderline personality disorder, dyslexia, and cognitive impairment, but as yet the supporting evidence for these uses remains exceedingly preliminary.

Other Conditions: Other proposed uses of fish oils with some support include asthma, Raynaud's phenomenon (abnormal sensitivity of hands and feet to cold), chronic fatigue syndrome, cystic fibrosis, osteoporosis, reducing the risk of prostate cancer, and preventing weight loss during cancer chemotherapy.

DHA is important for normal development and functioning of the brain and retina in the fetus and in infants. For this reason, pregnant or nursing mothers may benefit from supplementation. DHA is also often added to formula for premature infants and some regular infant formulas and foods. Omega-3s may also reduce the risk of premature delivery in pregnant women.

The balance of current evidence suggests that fish oil is not effective for migraine headaches, multiple sclerosis, psoriasis, male infertility and enhancing immunity in people with HIV.

Pet Use: Fish oil supplements are commonly given to pets to help maintain their coats and skin. (For more information, see "Joint-Care Supplements: Glucosamine, Chondroitin, and MSM," page 76, volume 1, and "Multivitamin/Multimineral Supplements," page 380.)

Quality Concerns and Product Testing

Because omega-3 fatty acids are obtained from natural sources, levels in supplements can vary, depending on the source and method of processing. Contamination has also been an issue because fish can accumulate toxins such as mercury, dioxins, and PCBs. Mercury can damage the nervous system, particularly in a fetus. Dioxins and polychlorinated biphenyls (PCBs) may be carcinogens at low levels of exposure over time and may have other deleterious effects. The freshness of the oil is also an important consideration because rancid fish oils have an extremely unpleasant odor and may not be as effective. Neither the FDA nor any other federal or state agency routinely tests fish or marine oil supplements for quality prior to sale.

ConsumerLab.com, as part of its mission to independently evaluate products that affect health, wellness, and nutrition, purchased many dietary supplements sold in the U.S. claiming to contain EPA and/or DHA and tested them for their levels of EPA and DHA, mercury, PCBs, and signs of decomposition. Some of the products were tested for dioxins at the request of their manufacturers. Among the products purchased and tested, the majority was for use by people; a few were for pets. Most of the supplements were softgels, but some were liquids and one came in packet form.

Test Findings

Tests of omega-3 fatty acid supplements showed that all but two were fresh and contained their claimed amounts of EPA and DHA, key omega-3 fatty acids.

None of the products were found to contain detectable levels of mercury (more than 10 parts per billion [ppb]). By comparison, mercury levels in fish generally range from 10 ppb to 1,000 ppb, depending on the fish (see ConsumerTips™ for Buying and Using, page 503). In addition, none of the products contained unsafe levels of PCBs. PCBs have been found in several fish, including farm-raised salmon. Several of the products (footnoted) were additionally tested for dioxins, which can be found in some fish. However, none of these supplements contained unsafe levels of dioxins. (See the appropriate section in "ConsumerLab.com's Testing Methods and Standards," page 666.)

The lack of contaminants in the supplements has several possible explanations: (1) the use of species of fish least likely to accumulate mercury; (2) the fact that most mercury is found in fish meat, not oil; and (3) distillation processes that can remove contaminants.

The two products that failed the testing had the following problems. Garden of Life® (Formulated by Dr. Jordan S. Rubin) Olde World Icelandic Cod Liver Oil™ (Lemon Mint Flavor), a liquid product, was spoiled (indicated by elevated amounts of both peroxide [recent spoilage] and anisidine [longer-term spoilage]).

EHP Products Salmon Oil, a soft-gel supplement, contained only 53% of its claimed EPA. This product is sold for human use and marketed for pet use.

The 16 products that were selected for testing and a summary of the results are listed alphabetically in Test Results for Omega-3 Supplements. Also included in the list are 26 other products (indicated with an asterisk) that have met the same criteria through CL's Voluntary Certification Program (see Selection and Testing, page 25, volume 1).

ConsumerTips™ for Buying and Using

Food Sources: You may want to consider getting omega-3 fatty acids directly from fish. For the general population, the American Heart Association (AHA) recommends at least two 3-oz servings of fish a week. Fatty fish have the highest levels of omega-3 fatty acids.

<table>
<tr><td colspan="2">

Food Sources of Omega-3 Fatty Acids

</td></tr>
<tr>
<td>

Anchovies
Bluefish
Carp
Catfish
Halibut
Herring
Lake Trout
</td>
<td>

Mackerel
Pompano
Salmon*
Striped Sea Bass
White Tuna (Albacore)**
Whitefish
</td>
</tr>
<tr><td colspan="2">

Source: U.S. Department of Agriculture, Agricultural Research Service. 2001.
* Farmed salmon may contain more PCBs than other salmon.
** May contain an excessive amount of mercury.
</td></tr>
</table>

Total amounts of omega-3s vary among fish, but ones listed in Food Sources of Omega-3 Fatty Acids are all good sources. A three-ounce serving of canned albacore white tuna, for example, contains about 2.5 grams of fat, about 30% of which is EPA (200 mg) and DHA (500 mg). Light tuna contains less than half the omega-3 oils of white tuna.

Levels of pollutants, such as mercury, tend to be higher in long-lived, larger fish, particularly shark, swordfish, king mackerel, and tilefish. These fish tend to average about 1,000 ppb (parts per billion) of mercury—the FDA limit for human consumption—although most other fish tend to have about one-tenth to one-third of this amount. Eating a fish with 1,000 ppb of mercury is not necessarily toxic, but such fish should not be consumed by young children and pregnant or nursing women, or by anyone on a regular basis. The Environmental Protection Agency (EPA) has also advised that fresh-water fish may contain more mercury than commercially caught fish and advises that "If you are pregnant or could become pregnant, are nursing a baby, or feeding a young child, limit consumption of fish caught by family and friends to one meal (about 6 ounces) of fish per week." The same limit is recommended for albacore (white) tuna, as it may contain excessive levels of mercury. A recent study has also shown that some farm-raised salmon contain higher levels of PCBs than wild salmon.

If you are concerned about mercury and other potential contaminants, concentrated fish oil products may be a better choice, provided that they contain the claimed amount of oils and meet other quality parameters.

Eggs fortified with DHA are also now available in the U.S. and claim to contain 150 mg of DHA in each egg, which is about the amount found in 3 ounces of salmon. Chickens producing these eggs are typically fed algal DHA. Algal DHA has been approved as a food ingredient, so that foods and beverages can be fortified with DHA. Because some formula-fed infants may not be converting enough ALA to DHA, some formulas are also now available with DHA, which has been added to formulas for premature infants for many years.

Supplements: When buying supplements containing EPA and DHA, keep in mind that products vary significantly in terms of the amounts and ratios of EPA and DHA. Many products made from menhaden and other small fish have a ratio of EPA to DHA of 1.5; that is, a capsule claiming 1 gram (1,000 mg) of fish oil provides 180 mg of EPA and 120 mg of DHA, or slightly less than one-third of the fish oil comes in the form of omega-3s. However, a more concentrated product may contain twice that amount of both EPA and DHA.

Products made from other types of fish or marine sources can contain a variety of amounts and ratios of EPA and DHA. Some salmon oil products, for example, claim to contain more DHA than EPA and products made just from algal oil will contain only DHA. With a more concentrated product, one may be able to take fewer capsules of the same size. Semi-synthetic (ester) forms of EPA and DHA are also available and are thought to be as active as the natural (triacylglycerol) forms, although a preliminary study in rats suggests that their actions may not be identical.

Many products also contain vitamin E or other antioxidants to stabilize the oils and prevent them from becoming rancid.

Your daily intake should be based on your reason for taking fish oil and the amount that you are already getting from your diet.

Omega-3 vs. Omega-6 Fatty Acids: Some experts suggest that the American diet contains too little omega-3 fatty acids and too much of another essential fatty acid family called the omega-6 fatty acids. The typical ratio of omega-6s to omega-3s in the American diet is thought to be as high as 14:1 (14 grams of omega 6s for every gram of omega-3s). These experts suggest that a ratio of no more than 3:1 (3 grams of omega-6s for every 1 gram of omega-3) may be preferable. However, the evidence for this recommendation is sketchy at best.

A typical dose of fish oil is 6 to 12 grams daily. However, EPA and DHA represent only part of the total oil in fish and their levels vary among products. For most therapeutic uses of omega-3s, the daily dosage of total EPA and DHA tested in studies has ranged from 3 to 6 grams daily. Higher dosages have been tried by some researchers, especially for the treatment of schizophrenia, Raynaud's phenomenon, and lupus.

The American Heart Association recommends fish oil capsules for patients with extremely high triglycerides (greater than 1,000 mg/dl), who have not responded well to other treatments. In treating patients with high triglycerides, about 5 grams of combined EPA and DHA is recommended daily. As little as one gram daily of combined EPA and DHA may be adequate for reducing risk of a recurrent heart attack.

For pregnant and nursing women, the recommended dose of DHA, from either supplements or fish, is 100 to 200 mg a day.

Although there is no official recommended intake for omega-3s in healthy people, some experts have said that a total intake of about 650 milligrams (with at least 220 mg coming from each DHA and EPA) a day is a good goal. The remaining 200+ mg can come from either DHA or EPA.

Fish oils are best tolerated when taken with meals, and should be taken in divided doses; that is, divide the dose in half and take twice daily, or in thirds and take three times a day.

Concerns and Cautions

Although fish oil supplements are generally considered safe, you should take the following information into consideration before you buy:

The most common side effects are fishy-smelling burps and diarrhea.

Up to about 20 grams of fish oil can be well tolerated by most adults. However, such high amounts may not be beneficial and the FDA recommends that consumers not exceed more than a total of 3 grams a day of EPA and DHA omega-3 fatty acids, with no more than 2 grams a day from a dietary supplement.

Cod liver oil is not a good substitute for fish oil supplements because it is high in vitamins A and D. Also, these vitamins can be toxic, so make sure that you do not exceed safe levels (see pages 386 and 390 for Tolerable Upper Intake Levels [UL] of vitamins A and D).

The only significant safety concerns regarding fish oil involve its apparent blood-thinning effect. For this reason, people with bleeding disorders such as hemophilia; those taking strong prescription blood thinners, such as Coumadin (warfarin) or heparin; and those expecting to undergo surgery should use fish oils under a physician's care only.

Contrary to earlier reports, fish oil does not appear to adversely affect blood sugar levels in people with diabetes.

Test Results for Omega-3 Supplements

Product (label info: EPA/DHA/ Unit, dosing)‡ Daily serving (Mf. suggested)of EPA and DHA Manufacturer (Mf) or distributor (Dist)	Test Results			
	Approved or not approved	Contained claimed amount of EPA and DHA	Acceptable level of mercury and PCBs, and safe level of dioxins	Freshness
Softgels and Packets				
Advocare® OMEGAPLEX® Omega-3 Fatty Acid (300 mg EPA, 200 mg DHA/ softgel, 3/day) Daily: EPA: 900 mg and DHA: 600 mg Dist: Advocare International	approved	✔	✔	✔
Allergy Research Group® Super EPA Fish Oil Concentrate (360 mg EPA, 240 mg DHA/softgel, 2–6/day) Daily: EPA: 720–2160 mg and DHA: 480–144 mg Dist: Allergy Research Group	approved	✔	✔	✔

continued

Product (label info.)	Test Results			
	Approval	Contained claimed	Acceptable levels	Freshness
Berkley & Jensen™ Fish Oil Concentrate 1,000 mg with Omega-3 Fatty Acids (150 mg EPA, 100 mg DHA/softgel, 3–6/day) Daily: EPA: 450–900 mg and DHA: 300–600 mg Dist: BJWC	approved	✔	✔	✔
Cardiovascular Research Ltd MaxEPA™ Marine Lipid Concentrate (180 mg EPA, 120 mg DHA/softgel, 2/day) Daily: EPA: 360 mg and DHA: 240 mg Dist: Cardiovascular Research Ltd	approved	✔	✔	✔
Carlson® Super Omega-3 Fish Oils 1,000 mg (300 mg EPA, 200 mg DHA/softgel, 1/day)* Daily: EPA: 300 mg and DHA: 200 mg Dist: Carlson Div. of J.R. Carlson	approved	✔	✔	✔

Product (label info.)	Test Results			
	Approval	Contained claimed	Acceptable levels	Freshness
Coromega™ omega–3 Fish Oil (350 mg EPA, 230 mg DHA/packet, 1/day)* Daily: EPA: 350 mg and DHA: 230 mg Dist: ERBL, Inc	approved	✔	✔†	✔
CVS® pharmacy Natural Fish Oil Concentrate 1000 mg (180 mg EPA, 120 mg DHA/ softgel, 3/day)* Daily: EPA: 540 mg and DHA: 360 mg Dist: CVS	approved	✔	✔	✔
GNC Preventive Nutrition® Omega Complex (60 mg EPA, 40 mg DHA/ softgel, 3/day)* Daily: EPA: 180 mg and DHA: 120 mg Dist: General Nutrition Corporation	approved	✔	✔	✔

continued

Product (label info.)	Test Results			
	Approval	Contained claimed	Acceptable levels	Freshness
Health From The Sun The Total EFA™, Flax, Fish, Borage 1200 mg (72 mg EPA, 48 mg DHA/ softgel, 3/day)*[3] Daily: EPA: 216 mg and DHA: 144 mg Mf: Arkopharma, LLC	approved; also approved for flaxseed and borage oils	✔	✔	✔
Kirkland Signature™ Natural Fish Oil Concentrate 1,000 mg with Omega-3 Fatty Acids (150 mg EPA, 100 mg DHA/ softgel, 2/day) Daily: EPA: 300 mg and DHA: 200 mg Dist: Costco Wholesale Corporation	approved	✔	✔	✔

Product (label info.)	Test Results			
	Approval	Contained claimed	Acceptable levels	Freshness
Metagenics® EPA-DHA 6:1 TG™ 500mg Concentrated EPA, Optimal Absorption (50 mg EPA, 60–100 mg DHA/ softgel, 1–6/day) Daily: EPA: 500–3000 mg and DHA: 60–600 mg Dist: Metagenics Inc	approved	✔	✔	✔
Natrol Omega-3 Purified Fish Oil (180 mg EPA, 120 mg DHA/ softgel, 2–4/day) Daily: EPA: 360–720 mg and DHA: 240–480 mg Mf: Natrol, Inc.	approved	✔	✔	✔
Nature's Bounty® Cold Water Salmon Oil 1,000 mg (80 mg EPA, 120 mg DHA/softgel, 4/day)* Daily: EPA: 320 mg and DHA: 480 mg Mf: Nature's Bounty Inc	approved	✔	✔	✔

continued

Product (label info.)	Test Results			
	Approval	Contained claimed	Acceptable levels	Freshness
Nature's Bounty® Natural Fish Oil 1,000 mg Cholesterol Free (180 mg EPA, 120 mg DHA/softgel, 3/day)* Daily: EPA: 540 mg and DHA: 360 mg Mf: Nature's Bounty Inc	approved	✔	✔	✔
Nordic Naturals Ultimate™ Omega, lemon taste (325 mg EPA, 225 mg DHA/ softgel, 2/day)* Daily: EPA: 650, DHA: 450 Mf: Nordic Naturals, Inc.	approved	✔	✔†	✔
Nutrilite® Omega 3 Complex (65 mg EPA, 45 mg DHA/ softgel, 1–3/day)* Daily: EPA: 65– 195 mg and DHA: 45–135 mg Dist: Access Business Group International LLC	approved	✔	✔	✔

Product (label info.)	Test Results			
	Approval	Contained claimed	Acceptable levels	Freshness
OLAY™ Vitamins essential balanced omega 3/6™, Enteric Coated for Better Digestion (93.6 mg EPA, 187 mg DHA/ enteric-coated softgel, 1/day)* Daily: EPA: 93.6 mg and DHA: 187.2 mg Dist: Pharmavite LLC	approved	✔	✔†	✔
OmegaBrite™ 100% Natural Advanced Omega 3 Formula, 500 mg (375 mg EPA, 55 mg DHA/softgel, 3/day)* Daily: EPA: 1125 mg and DHA: 165 mg Dist: Omega Natural Health	approved	✔	✔†	✔
Origin® Natural Fish Oil Concentrate 1,000 mg (180 mg EPA, 120 mg DHA/ softgel, 3/day)* Daily: EPA: 540 mg and DHA: 360 mg Dist: Target Corporation	approved	✔	✔	✔

continued

Product (label info.)	Test Results			
	Approval	Contained claimed	Acceptable levels	Freshness
PhytoPharmica® ESKIMO-3® Naturally Stable Fish Oil® (70 mg EPA, 42 mg DHA/softgel, 3–9/ day)*[4] Daily: PA: 210–630 mg and DHA: 125–375 mg Mf: Cardinova International	approved	✔	✔	✔
Puritan's Pride® Cholesterol Free Fish Oil 1,200 mg (216 mg EPA, 144 mg DHA/ softgel, 3/day)* Daily: EPA: 648 mg and DHA: 432 mg Mf: Puritan's Pride, Inc.	approved	✔	✔	✔
Puritan's Pride® Cholesterol Free Natural Fish Oil EPA 1,000 mg (180 mg EPA, 120 mg DHA/softgel, 3/day)* Daily: EPA: 540 mg and DHA: 360 mg Mf: Puritan's Pride, Inc.	approved	✔	✔	✔

Product (label info.)	Test Results			
	Approval	Contained claimed	Acceptable levels	Freshness
Puritan's Pride® Triple Omega 3-6-9 Flax, Fish & Borage Oil (120 mg EPA, 80 mg DHA/softgel, 1–2/day)* Daily: EPA: 120–240 mg and DHA: 80–150 mg Mf: Puritan's Pride, Inc.	approved	✔	✔	✔
Rexall® Flax, Fish, Borage Oil (120 mg EPA, 80 mg DHA/softgel, 1–2/day)* Daily: EPA: 120–240 mg and DHA: 80–160 mg Mf: Rexall, Inc.	approved	✔	✔	✔
Sav-on Osco by Albertsons™ Natural Fish Oil Concentrate 1,000 mg with Omega-3 Fatty Acids (180 mg EPA, 120 mg DHA/softgel, 3/day) Daily: EPA: 540 mg and DHA: 360 mg Dist: Albertsons Inc.	approved	✔	✔	✔

continued

Product Reviews: Special Ingredients

Product (label info.)	Test Results			
	Approval	Contained claimed	Acceptable levels	Freshness
Source Naturals® Neuromins™ DHA 100 mg (100 mg DHA/softgel, 1–2/day) Daily: EPA: 0 mg and DHA: 100–200 mg Dist: Source Naturals, Inc.	approved	✔	✔	✔
Spring Valley Fish Oil 1,200 mg (216 mg EPA, 144 mg DHA/softgel, 3/day)* Daily: EPA: 648 mg and DHA: 432 mg Mf: Nature's Bounty, Inc.	approved	✔	✔	✔
Sundown® Fish Oil 1,000 mg (180 mg EPA, 120 mg DHA/softgel, 2–6/day)* Daily: EPA: 360–1080 mg and DHA: 240–720 mg Dist: Rexall Sundown, Inc.	approved	✔	✔	✔

Product (label info.)	Test Results			
	Approval	Contained claimed	Acceptable levels	Freshness
Swanson EPAs Superior Essential Fatty Acids ecOmega™ EPA/ DHA (180 mg EPA, 120 mg DHA/ softgel, 2/day) Daily: EPA: 360 mg and DHA: 240 mg Dist: Swanson Health Products	approved	✔	✔	✔
The Vitamin Shoppe™ Essential Oils & Fatty Acids EPA-DHA Omega-3 Fish Oil 500 (300 mg EPA, 200 mg DHA/ softgel, 1–2/day)* Daily: EPA: 300–600 mg and DHA: 200–400 mg Dist: The Vitamin Shoppe	approved	✔	✔†	✔
Triomega® Omega-3 (333.3 mg EPA, 167 mg DHA/softgel, 1/day)* Daily: EPA: 333.3 mg and DHA: 166.67 mg Dist: Inverness Medical, Inc.	approved	✔	✔†	✔

continued

Product (label info.)	Test Results			
	Approval	Contained claimed	Acceptable levels	Freshness
Vitamin World® Cholesterol Free Fish Oil 1,200 mg (216 mg EPA, 144 mg DHA/ softgel, 3/day)* Daily: EPA: 648 mg and DHA: 432 mg Mf: Vitamin World	approved	✔	✔	✔
Vitamin World® Naturally Inspired™ Omega-3 Fish Oil 1,000 mg Cholesterol-Free (180 mg EPA, 120 mg DHA/ softgel, 3/day)* Daily: EPA: 540 mg and DHA: 360 mg Mf: Vitamin World	approved	✔	✔	✔
Vitamin World® Naturally Inspired™ Super EPA Natural Fish Oil 1,000 mg Cholesterol-Free (300 mg EPA, 200 mg DHA/ softgel, 3/day)* Daily: EPA: 900 mg and DHA: 600 mg Mf: Vitamin World	approved	✔	✔	✔

Product (label info.)	Test Results			
	Approval	Contained claimed	Acceptable levels	Freshness
Vitamin World® Triple Omega 3-6-9 Flax, Fish & Borage Oil (120 mg EPA, 80 mg DHA/softgel, 3/day)* Daily: EPA: 360 mg and DHA: 240 mg Mf: Vitamin World	approved	✔	✔	✔
Whole Foods™ Molecularly Distilled Fish Oil (Concentrated Omega-3 EFAs) 1,000 mg (180 mg EPA, 120 mg DHA/softgel, 1–3/day) Daily: EPA: 180–540 mg and DHA: 120–360 mg Dist: Whole Foods Market	approved	✔	✔	✔

continued

Product (label info.)	Test Results			
	Approval	Contained claimed	Acceptable levels	Freshness
Zone Perfect® Omega 3 Molecular Distilled Fish Oil & Vitamin E 1,000 mg (160 mg EPA) (107 mg DHA) Cholesterol Free (160 mg EPA, 107 mg DHA/ softgel, 2–4/day) discontinued Daily: EPA: 320–640 mg and DHA: 214–428 mg Dist: Zone Perfect Nutrition Co	approved	✔	✔	✔
Liquids				
Carlson® Norwegian Cod Liver Oil (460–500 mg EPA, 500–550 mg DHA/ 5 mL liquid, 1/day or more)* Daily: EPA: 460–550 at 5 mL/ day and DHA: 500–550 at 5 mL/ day Dist: J.R. Carlson Laboratories, Inc.	approved[1]	✔	✔	✔

Product (label info.)	Test Results			
	Approval	Contained claimed	Acceptable levels	Freshness
Garden of Life® (Formulated by Dr. Jordan S. Rubin) Olde World Icelandic Cod Liver Oil™ Lemon Mint Flavor (320 mg EPA, 453 mg DHA/5 mL liquid, 1–3/day for adults, 0.5–1.5/day for children) Daily: EPA: (Adults) 320–960 mg; (Children) 160–480 mg and DHA: (Adults) 453–1359 mg; (Children) 226.5–679.5 mg Dist: Garden of Life	*not* approved[2]	✔	✔	failed
Pet Supplements				
EHP Products Salmon Oil Dietary Supplement, 1,000 mg (180 mg EPA, 120 mg DHA/ softgel, 1/day)** Daily: EPA: 360 mg and DHA: 240 mg Dist: EHP Products Inc	*not* approved	Contained 53% of claimed EPA	✔	✔

continued

Product Reviews: Special Ingredients

Product (label info.)	Test Results			
	Approval	Contained claimed	Acceptable levels	Freshness
DermCare® Veterinary Formulas Dietary Supplement Capsules with Omega-3 (Large Breeds) for Dogs (360 mg EPA, 240 mg DHA/ softgel, 1–3/day) Daily: EPA: 180–540 mg and DHA: 120–360 mg Dist: HAVA Pet Products	approved	✔	✔	✔
Skin Formula 3V Caps™ for medium and large breeds of dogs (180 mg EPA, 120 mg DHA/ softgel, 1–2/day) Daily: EPA: 180–360 mg DHA: 120–240 mg Dist: DVM Pharmaceuticals	approved	✔	✔	✔

*Tested through CL's Voluntary Certification Program before, at the time of, or after the initial review.

✔ Check indicates the results met the criteria listed in the column heading.

‡ See also "More Brand Information," page 675.

**This product is sold for human use but is also marketed for use by pets.

† Product participated in optional dioxin testing at the request of its manufacturer/distributor through CL's Voluntary Certification Program. Safe level of dioxins found.

[1] Product label suggests taking 1 or more teaspoonfuls per day. Tolerable Upper Intake Level (UL) for vitamin A would be exceeded if more than 8 teaspoonfuls were taken daily by adults or more than 1 to 2 teaspoonfuls taken daily by children.

[2] Tolerable Upper Intake Level for vitamin A would be exceeded if maximum suggested dose was taken by adults or children.

[3] An earlier version of this product did not pass this review. It had the lot number 8030 and expiration date September 2006.

[4] CL was informed in August 2006 that this product is no longer sold under the PhytoPharmica brand but is now sold under the Enzymatic Therapy brand.

Probiotic Supplements (Including *Lactobacillus acidophilus, Bifidobacterium,* and Others)

Probiotic products contain helpful bacteria and/or yeasts that assist in balancing the levels of indigenous microorganisms in the human body. Probiotics are available in varied forms such as yogurt and other cultured milk foods, capsules, tablets, beverages, and powders. *Probiotics* should not be confused with *prebiotics*, which are complex sugars (such as inulin and other fructo-oligosaccharides) that are ingested as fuel for bacteria already present in the gastrointestinal tract. Prebiotics and probiotics are sometimes combined in the same product and termed *syn*biotics.

The normal human gastrointestinal tract contains hundreds of different species of bacteria, referred to as intestinal flora. When the normal balance of these bacteria is disturbed by illness or antibiotic treatment, the most common effect is diarrhea. Probiotics work by recolonizing the small intestine and crowding out disease-causing bacteria, thereby restoring balance to the intestinal flora. They may also produce substances that inhibit pathogenic bacteria, compete for nutrients with them, and stimulate the body's own immune system.

Saccharomyces boulardii (a probiotic yeast) and the bacteria *Enterococcus faecium* and *Lactobacillus* have been clinically proven to prevent antibiotic-caused diarrhea. Successful clinical trials have also been conducted using *Lactobacillus* alone or in combination with *Bifidobacterium* and *Saccharomyces* species to treat *H. pylori* infection (a causative agent of stomach ulcers). A strain of *Bifidobacterium* or a combination of *Lactobacillus, Bifidobacterium,* and *Streptococcus* species has been used to successfully treat symptoms of irritable bowel syndrome (IBS), although studies with other strains have not shown a benefit. *Lactobacillus GG* (a strain of *L. rhamnosus*) and *Lactobacillus reuteri* have been shown to reduce the duration of diarrhea due to certain infections in infants and young children.

Unfortunately, studies using probiotics (*Lactobacillus, Bifidobacterium, Streptococcus,* and *Saccharomyces* species) to treat traveler's diarrhea have not shown definitive results. The effectiveness of individual probiotic species for traveler's diarrhea may vary depending on the travel destination. Although the evidence is not clear-cut, probiotics have been studied as a treatment for many other conditions and their symptoms including lactose intolerance, respiratory and GI problems resulting from cystic fibrosis, HIV-related diarrhea, Crohn's disease, ulcerative colitis pouchitis, cancer prevention, high blood cholesterol, tuberculosis, eczema, acne, canker sores, dental cavities, milk allergies, common colds, hay fever, vaginal and urinary tract infections, enhanced immune system activity, and prevention of respiratory infections in children. See ConsumerTips™ for Buying and Using, page 527, for dosage information.

Quality Concerns and Product Testing

Neither the FDA nor any other federal or state agency routinely tests probiotics for quality prior to sale. However, quality issues for probiotic supplements can include the following: The viability of organisms in the product—how many organisms are alive (in the case of active cultures) or can "come alive" from their inactive state when purchased and used? Some products make no claim at all and others claim only the amount at the time of manufacture. Lack of contaminating organisms—the product should contain the bacteria and/or yeast that it claims on the label while potentially pathogenic microorganisms and other microbial contaminants should not be present. Enteric protection of the product—some types of bacteria cannot survive as they pass through stomach acid and into the small intestine where the bacteria would grow (see ConsumerTips™ for Buying and Using, page 527, for more information). Ideally, the product should contain bacteria that research shows can survive passage through the stomach or it should be enteric coated if they cannot survive the stomach acid. Products in tablets (with and without enteric coatings) should also be able to properly disintegrate so as to release the probiotic bacteria and not pass through the body intact.

ConsumerLab.com, as part of its mission to independently evaluate products that affect health, wellness, and nutrition, purchased many leading probiotic products sold in the U.S. and Canada and tested them to determine whether they 1) possessed the claimed amount of viable bacteria listed on the label and at least 1 billion live organisms per suggested daily serving, 2) were free of contamination with other yeast, mold, or types of bacteria with disease-causing potential, and 3) disintegrated properly (if in tablet form) so that their contents would be released, or if enteric-coated, their contents would be released after passing through the stomach. (See "ConsumerLab.com's Testing Methods and Standards," page 667.)

Test Findings

ConsumerLab selected 13 probiotic products sold in the U.S. and/or Canada. Only eight of these were found to contain at least 1 billion organisms per daily dose (a generally recommended minimum) and any higher amounts that they may have claimed on their labels. An additional six products tested through CL's Voluntary Certification Program also met these criteria. Some products provided several billion or tens of billions of organisms per day.

Four products were found to provide less than one billion viable organisms in a daily serving. It is possible that products with such low levels may not work or work as well as products with more viable organisms. Some clinical studies have shown that products with even tens of millions of live bacteria may be ineffective. Products with less than one billion viable organisms were: Advocare® Probiotic Restore™ claimed that two to four capsules provided 2 to 4 billion organisms. A dose of two capsules did not provide 1 billion, although four capsules did. DDS® Acidophilus with FOS claimed to provide 2 billion organisms at the time it was made, but it had less than 1 billion when tested. Nature's Secret Ultimate Probiotic claimed 4 billion at the time it was made, but had less than 1 billion when tested. Rite Aid Acidophilus didn't state an amount of organisms, but a daily serving (1 capsule) contained only 30 million organisms.

A fifth product, Flora Source™, had the minimum 1 billion organisms per daily serving, but did not contain the 30 billion guaranteed to be in the product at the time it was made.

When a product indicates that its claimed number of probiotic organisms reflects the amount "at the time of manufacture," it means that the company is not guaranteeing how much you'll get when you buy it. It's hard to say if this practice suggests a potential problem, as some products labeled this way did contain their listed amounts while others did not. Products that do not limit their claims to the time of manufacture should be expected to deliver the amounts on their labels—although not all do.

Pet Use: ConsumerLab.com also tested probiotic supplements marketed for use by pets. Among the three products selected, one was contaminated with mold and did not contain its listed amount of probiotic organisms. Another provided only 10 million organisms per day. Only one product contained a large dose of viable organisms—2.3 billion.

All tablet products disintegrated properly so that their organisms would be released in the body. An enteric-coated supplement in "pearl" form passed special testing that confirmed its ability to pass through the stomach and deliver its bacteria to the intestine. See "ConsumeLab.com's Testing Methods and Standards," page 667, for more information about the testing and criteria.

Listed alphabetically in Test Results for Probiotic Supplements are the Test Results for 22 supplements—19 marketed for human use and 3 for use by pets. ConsumerLab.com selected 16 of the products. Six others (each indicated with an asterisk) were tested at the request of their manufacturers/distributors through CL's Voluntary Certification Program and are included for having passed testing.

ConsumerTips™ for Buying and Using

Properly labeled probiotic supplements will list the types of bacteria and/or yeast that are present. Names of the organisms should be listed in italics, with the genus name capitalized and listed first. The genus name may also be abbreviated with its first letter (e.g., *Lactobacillus acidophilus* or *L. acidophilus*).

The species most commonly seen in probiotics and that have been tested in laboratory and clinical studies are *Lactobacillus acidophilus, L. bulgaricus, L. casei, L. gasseri, L. plantarum, Bifidobacterium bifidum, B. lactis, B. longum, Enterococcus faecium,* and *Saccharomyces boulardii* (a yeast). Other species that can be used as probiotics but have less accompanying research are *L. johnsonii, L. reuteri, L. rhamnosus, B. breve, B. infantis, E. faecalis,* and *Streptococcus salivarius*. Some probiotic bacterial strains have been patented and are accompanied by substantial research into their effects. *L. casei GG* (a strain of *Lactobacillus rhamnosus* found in Culturelle capsules), *L. casei* in Actimel (Dannon), and LC1 (Nestle) are three examples. Some research has shown that it may be more effective to take a probiotic supplement that contains a mixture of bacterial strains rather than a single bacterial species.

While many products make claims regarding the number of organisms in the product, these typically refer to the numbers at the time of manufacture—which can be very different from the amount still viable at the time of purchase. Exposure to heat, moisture, and oxygen can all negatively affect probiotic survival, so the expiration date is especially important to note.

Some products have an enteric coating because certain probiotic bacteria need protection to survive exposure to stomach acid. Most *Lactobacillus, Bifidobacterium,* and *Streptococcus* species do not need enteric coating, as they can safely pass through the stomach.

Some bacteria naturally sporulate ("hibernate" within a protective coating) when they are exposed to harsh conditions, and some researchers postulate that sporulated bacteria are more resistant to the harsh conditions found in the GI tract. Consequently, another delivery method is to manufacture probiotics in the form of bacterial spores—this is most often used for bacteria of the genus *Bacillus* and *Lactobacillus sporogenes.*

L. bulgaricus and *S. thermophilus,* as well as *Leuconostoc* and *Lactococcus* species, cannot survive passage through the stomach. These bacteria are commonly found in yogurt because they are used as starters for dairy products. Although they cannot colonize the intestinal tract, they may still have benefits: *S. thermophilus,* for example, produces large quantities of lactic acid, which may limit the growth of unfriendly bacteria and help in the prevention and treatment of diarrhea. Yogurts and other dairy products specifically marketed as probiotics will often have additional species added that can withstand the stomach acid.

Probiotics are measured in terms of the number of live organisms per dose and stated as units or colony-forming units (CFU). The recommended intake for probiotic supplements is 1 billion to 10 billion units per day. These amounts may be written on the label as "1×10^9" or "10^9" for 1 billion units, and "1×10^{10}" or "10^{10}" for 10 billion units. The types and number of organisms taken as probiotics depend on the diagnosed use.

For the treatment of antibiotic-related diarrhea, it is recommended to start taking probiotic supplements as soon as symptoms appear. However, if symptoms persist for several days, see a physician. Probiotics can be taken starting the first day of oral antibiotic treatment and continued for 2 weeks after the end of antibiotic therapy. It may be advisable to take probiotics and antibiotics at least 2 hours apart to reduce any possibility that the antibiotic might kill the probiotic organisms. For rotaviral diarrhea in infants and children up to age 3, doses of up to 10 billion cells of *Lactobacillus GG* and *Lactobacillus reuteri* may significantly reduce diarrheal infection.

For treating vaginal bacterial infections, vaginal suppositories containing approximately 1 billion *Lactobacillus* organisms are typically used.

For irritable bowel syndrome (IBS), 1 billion cells daily of *Bifidobacterium infantis* in a malted drink for eight weeks has been shown to reduce abdominal pain, bloating, and bowel movement difficulty, but it does not reduce the frequency of bowel movements. A combination product of species including *Bifidobacterium, Lactobacillus,* and *Streptococcus* has also helped with IBS. (Studies with *Lactobacillus GG, Lactobacillus plantarum,* and *Lactobacillus salivarius* have not shown benefit with IBS.)

To gain probiotic benefits from yogurt or other dairy foods, look for products labeled "contains live cultures" or "active cultures." Some yogurts will state the species of bacteria they contain.

It is advisable to keep probiotics out of heat and light. After being opened, they should also be kept out of moisture to prevent organisms from becoming activated and then dying. Although not always required, it is advisable to keep probiotic products refrigerated.

Concerns and Cautions

There are no known safety issues with probiotic bacteria at appropriate doses in healthy people, but occasionally some people notice a temporary increase in digestive gas.

In a few cases among severely ill or immunocompromised individuals, probiotic use has caused bacteremia (presence of bacteria in the blood) or pathological infections resulting in severe illness. However, HIV-positive adults have taken probiotics for up to 3 weeks without side effects. There is a case report of an individual having an allergic reaction when exposed to foods containing inulin. Inulin is a *pre*biotic ingredient (often from chicory) added to some probiotic supplements.

Be aware that probiotic products may contain trace amounts of growth media residue left over from the manufacturing of probiotic cultures. This can be dairy (casein), soy, or even fish peptide residue, in trace amounts. The Food Allergen Labeling and Consumer Protection Act (FALCPA) requires that products made after January 1, 2006, with these potential allergens be labeled as such. Be aware that some products on the market may not carry this information, including any made prior to 2006, or by companies failing to comply with the law.

Test Results for Probiotic Supplements

Product (dose)‡ Daily: Listed number of probiotic organisms in maximum suggested daily serving Manufacturer (Mf) or Distributor (Dist)	Types of organisms claimed per unit (and amounts if specified)	Test Results	
		Contained listed amount of probiotic organisms**	Provided at least 1 billion bacteria per daily serving**
General			
Advocare® Probiotic Restore™ (2–4 capsules/day) Daily: 2–4 billion Dist: Advocare® International	L. acidophilus 0.5 billion, B. bifidum 0.5 billion	No	No (for 2 capsules) ✔ (for 4 capsules)
Culturelle® with Lactobacillus GG, All Natural (1 capsule/day) Daily: 10 billion[1] Dist: Allergy Research Group/ Nutricology	Lactobacillus GG	✔	✔

continued

Product Reviews: Special Ingredients

Product (dose)	Types of organisms claimed	Test Results	
		Contained listed amount	Provided 1 billion
DDS® Acidophilus with FOS (1 g of powder [1/4 tsp])/day) Daily: 2 billion[1] Dist: UAS Laboratories	L. acidophilus	No	No
Enzymatic Therapy™ Acidophilus Pearls™ (1 pearl/ day)* Daily: 1 billion Mf: Enzymatic Therapy, Inc.	L. acidophilus and B. longum	✔	✔
Flora Source™, 15 Billion Viable Cells per Capsule (2 capsules/day) Daily: 30 billion[1] Dist: MBA Company	B. bifidum, B. breve, B. infantis, B. lactis, B. longum, L. acidophilus, L. brevis, L. bulgaricus, L. casei, L. gasseri, L. paracasei, L. plantarum, L. rhamnosus, L. salivarius, L. lactis, Streptococcus thermophilus	No	✔

Product (dose)	Types of organisms claimed	Test Results	
		Contained listed amount	Provided 1 billion
Garden of Life® Primal Defense™ HSO™ Probiotic Formula (3 scoops powder/day, 0.9 g each) Daily: Not stated Mf: Garden of Life, Inc.	L. plantarum, B. bifidum, B. lactis, L. rhamnosus, B. breve, L. casei, L. brevis, L. salivarius, L. acidophilus, Bacillus subtilis, L. paracasei, B. longum	N/A	✔ Found 1.44 billion** per scoop (4.3 billion/ day)
Jarrow Formulas® Enhanced Probiotic System, Jarro-Dophilus EPS™ (1–2 capsules/day)* Daily: 4.4 billion–8.8 billion[1] Dist: Jarrow Formulas	L. rhamnosus R0011 680 million, L. casei R0215 680 million, L. plantarum R1012 340 million, L. acidophilus R0052 680 million, B. longum BB536 (morinaga strain) 680 million, B. breve R0070 340 million, Pediococcus acidilactici R1001 670 million, Lactococcus diacetylactis R0100 330 million	✔	✔
Kal® Acidophilus ProBiotic-5, 3 Billion Viable Organisms, 5 Strains (1 capsule/day) Daily: 3 billion[1] Mf: Nutraceutical Corp.	L. acidophilus, Lactobacillus spp., L. bulgaricus, S. thermophilus, B. bifidum	✔	✔

continued

533

Product (dose)	Types of organisms claimed	Test Results	
		Contained listed amount	Provided 1 billion
Kyo-Dophilus® 1.5 Billion Live Cells per Capsule (2 capsules/ day)* Daily: 3 billion Mf: Wakunaga of America Co. Ltd	L. acidophilus Ks-13, B. bifidum G9-1 and B. longum MM-2	✔	✔
Nature's Secret Ultimate Probiotic 4-Billion™ (1 tablet/day) Daily: 4 billion[1] Dist: Nature's Secret	L. acidophilus, B. bifidum, L. rhamnosus, L. salivarius, B. infantis, B. longum, L. bulgaricus, L. plantarum, L. casei, L. paracasei, Streptococcus thermophilus, L. brevis, L. reuteri, L. lactis, L. SP lactis, L. fermentum, L. helveticus, Enterococcus faecium, L. keferi	No	No
Nature's Sunshine® Bifidophilus Flora Force®, 4 billion total microorganisms/ capsule / (2 capsules/day) Daily: 8 billion Dist: Nature's Sunshine Products, Inc.	L. rhamnosus 1.25 billion, L. casei 1 billion, L. acidophilus 1.25 billion, B. longum 0.5 billion	✔	✔

Product (dose)	Types of organisms claimed	Test Results	
		Contained listed amount	Provided 1 billion
Nature's Way® Primadophilus® Optima, 14 Probiotic Strains Plus NutraFlora®, 35 Billion CFU, Enteric-Coated (1 capsule/day)* Daily: 35 billion Dist: Nature's Way Products, Inc.	L. casei-108, B. longum-135, L. acidophilus-122, L. plantarum-119, L. rhamnosus-111, L. rhamnosus-114, B. breve-129, B. bifidum-132, Lactococcus lactis-136 [sic], Streptococcus thermophilus-110, B. infantis-116, L. bulgaricus-137, L. salivarius-118, L. helveticus-128	✔	✔
Nutravite Acidophilus Plus, Heat Resistant (2 capsules/day) Daily: 2.8 billion Dist: Nutravite Pharmaceutical Inc.	L. acidophilus, L. rhamnosus, and B. longum	✔	✔
PB 8® Pro-Biotic Acidophilus for Life™ (2 capsules/day) Daily: Amount not stated Dist: Nutrition Now® Inc.	L. acidophilus, L. plantarum, L. rhamnosus, L. casei, L. paracasei, L. salivarius, B. bifidum and B. longum[1]	N/A	✔

continued

Product (dose)	Types of organisms claimed	Test Results	
		Contained listed amount	Provided 1 billion
Pharmanex® ProBio PCC™ Live Probiotics (1 capsule/day)* Daily: Not stated Dist: Pharmanex, a division of NSE Products, Inc.	L. fermentum	N/A	✔ Found 1.2 billion** per capsule
Probiotic Gut Buddies® (1 capsule/day)* Daily: 2 billion Mf: Tishcon Corp.	B. longum ME 0.4 billion, L. rhamnosus ME 0.4 billion, L. acidophilus ME 1.2 billion	✔	✔
Rite Aid Acidophilus, Milk Free, Natural (1 capsule/day) Daily: amount not stated Dist: Rite Aid Corp.	L. acidophilus, B. bifidum and L. bulgaricus	N/A	No Found 30 million** per capsule
❦webber naturals™ Acidophilus with Bifidus, Non Dairy (3 capsules/day) Daily: 18 billion[1] Dist: wn pharmaceuticals, ltd.	L. rhamnosus 3 billion, L. paracasei 1.8 billion, L. acidophilus 0.6 billion, B. longum 0.6 billion	✔	✔

Product (dose)	Types of organisms claimed	Test Results	
		Contained listed amount	Provided 1 billion
Children's Products			
Natural Factors® Children's Acidophilus Natural Strawberry Flavor Powder (1–3 g powder/day) Daily: 2–6 billion[1] Dist: Natural Factors	L. rhamnosus 1.3 billion, B. infantis 0.4 billion, S. thermophilus 0.19 billion, L. acidophilus 0.10 billion, L. delbrueckii subsp. bulgaricus 0.01 billion	✔	✔
Pet Products			
Ark Naturals® Gentle Digest®, Prebiotics & Probiotics, for Dogs & Cats (3 capsules/day) Daily: 0.15 billion Mf: Gulf Coast Nutritionals, Inc.	Lactic acid bacillus 0.05 billion	No	No[†]
Mitomax™ Premium Probiotics for Pets (2 capsules/day) Daily: Not stated Dist: Imagilin Technology, LLC	Pediococcus acidilacticii and Saccharomyces boulardii	N/A	✔ Found 2.3 billion** per capsule (4.6 billion/day)

continued

537

Product Reviews: Special Ingredients

Product (dose)	Types of organisms claimed	Test Results	
		Contained listed amount	**Provided 1 billion**
Vita-Treat™ Acidophilus Plus Vitamins, Dog & Puppy Formula (2 capsules/day) Daily: Not stated Dist: Vita-Treat™	L. acidophilus, L. plantarum, L. casei, and L. bulgaricus	N/A	No Found only 10 million** per capsule (20 million/ day)

‡ See also "More Brand Information," page 675.

*Tested through CL's Voluntary Certification Program prior to, at time of, or after initial posting of this Product Review.

**Amounts shown are actual from testing. ConsumerLab.com allowed a margin of error in determining whether products met claims and minimums. For products noted above as providing less than 1 billion organisms, applying such a margin of error still yields a result below 1 billion.

† Product also contained microbial contamination (mold).

¹ Product label indicates that listed amount and/or types of bacteria relates to the "time of manufacture." Otherwise, products should be expected to contain listed ingredients at time of purchase before expiration date.

✔ Check indicates the results met the criteria listed in the column heading.

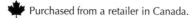 Purchased from a retailer in Canada.

SAMe

A naturally occurring compound, SAMe (also known as SAM-e, S-adenosyl-methionine, or S-adenosyl-L-methionine) is found in every cell in the body, where it's manufactured from the essential sulfur-containing amino acid methionine. Protein-rich foods are sources of this amino acid.

Although SAMe has many uses, it has primarily been shown to be effective as a treatment for osteoarthritis and associated joint pain, stiffness, and inflammation (see "Joint-Care Supplements," page 76, volume 1, for results for glucosamine, chondroitin, and MSM products). There is also some evidence for its short-term use in treating major depression (see separate review "St. John's Wort," page 286, volume 1, a supplement used for moderate and minor depression). Interestingly, the osteoarthritis application of SAMe was discovered during clinical trials for its use in depression.

Other potential applications include the treatment of fibromyalgia, liver disease, AIDS-related myelopathy, and attention-deficit/hyperactivity disorder (ADHD) in adults.

SAMe assists the body in producing a wide range of compounds, including neurotransmitters (such as dopamine and serotonin) and cartilage components (such as glycosaminoglycans). When natural SAMe levels are low, supplements may facilitate the production of these compounds.

Quality Concerns and Product Testing

SAMe is an expensive ingredient, so experts have been concerned about the actual quality and quantity of SAMe in supplements. Another concern is that SAMe can break down under certain circumstances resulting in less ingredient than what's stated on the label.

A stabilizing molecule is always added to SAMe products, often making it unclear as to the true weight of active SAMe because the weight of the inactive stabilizer may be included in the labeled amount. In fact, when first tested by ConsumerLab.com in 2000, nearly half of the products were found to contain significantly less SAMe than they claimed.

No government agency is responsible for routinely testing SAMe supplements for their contents or quality. However, ConsumerLab.

com independently evaluated several leading SAMe products to determine whether they possessed the SAMe amounts stated on their labels. All tablets and caplets were also tested to be sure that they would properly disintegrate (break apart). (See "ConsumerLab.com's Testing Methods and Standards," page 668.)

Test Findings

All eight of the SAMe supplements that CL selected for testing passed the evaluation. This is considerably better than results in 2003, in which one product was found with only 30% of its listed amount, and in 2000, when nearly half of the products were short on SAMe. All caplet and tablet products were able to disintegrate properly.

Listed alphabetically in Test Results for SAMe Supplements are the Test Results for ten SAMe products. ConsumerLab.com selected eight. Two (each indicated with an asterisk) were tested at the request of their manufacturer or distributor through CL's Voluntary Certification Program and are included for having passed testing. Also listed is one product similar to one that passed but sold under different a brand name.

ConsumerTips™ for Buying and Using

SAMe comes in different forms, depending on the compound used to stabilize it and prevent degradation. These compounds include tosylate, disulfate tosylate, disulfate ditosylate, and 1, 4-butanedisulfonate (Actimet™). They're usually written immediately after SAMe's chemical name. Because these added compounds weigh as much as the SAMe molecule itself, a tablet containing 200 mg of "S-adenosyl-methionine disulfate tosylate," for example, contains only 100 mg of SAMe. Most, but not all, labels make this clear. An accurate ingredient listing for SAMe in the Supplement Facts panel on a product should exclude the stabilizing compound, as does the dosage information below.

SAMe is absorbed from the intestine. Enteric-coated products, which aren't likely to break down in the stomach, are available. Consumers should choose these to prevent possible nausea and stomach upset.

Generally recommended daily doses of SAMe range from 200 to 800 mg, depending on the condition, its severity, and course of treatment.

For treating osteoarthritis, many experts recommend starting with a dose of 200 to 400 mg SAMe for the first day of therapy. Thereafter, 400 mg to 800 mg per day, taken in divided doses of 200 mg, is recommended. Losing weight and switching from high-impact to low-impact sports are also recommended for people with osteoarthritis.

For depression, doses ranging of 400 to 1,600 mg per day have been used.

For fibromyalgia, 800 mg per day is typically used.

For liver disease, higher doses of 1,200 mg to 1,600 mg per day have been used for treatment.

After starting SAMe supplementation, improvements may take anywhere from a few days to five weeks to become noticeable. The doses noted above are for SAMe taken orally. SAMe also has been taken by injection under medical supervision.

Concerns and Cautions

SAMe is generally considered safe when taken in appropriate doses, but be aware that it may occasionally cause nausea and stomach upset. Taking enteric-coated products, reducing the SAMe dosage, or taking it with meals can reduce these adverse effects.

Individuals with bipolar (manic-depressive) disorder should know that SAMe could trigger a manic phase. People taking standard antidepressants, including MAO inhibitors, SSRIs, and tricyclics should not take SAMe except on a physician's advice. Also, SAMe might help relieve the side effects of levodopa treatment (for Parkinson's disease), but it might also reduce its effectiveness over time. SAMe products aren't likely to help severe osteoarthritis, where cartilage has worn down so much that bone rubs against bone.

Test Results for SAMe Supplements

Product (label info: amount of SAMe, dose)‡ Daily amount of SAMe Manufacturer (Mf) or distributor (Dist)	Test Results		
	Approved or not approved	Contained claimed amount of key ingredient	Broke apart properly
Baywood PureChoice® SAMe S-Adenosyl-Methionine (100 mg/ tablet, 2–4/day) Daily: 200–400 mg SAMe enteric-coated Dist: Baywood	approved	✔	✔
Jarrow Formulas® Pharmaceutical Grade, Stabilized; Natural SAM-e 200; Full Potency; S-Adenosyl Methionine; 200 mg Elemental SAM-e from 400 mg SAM-e tosylate disulfate; (200 mg/tablet, 1–2/day) Daily: 200–400 mg SAMe enteric-coated Dist: Jarrow Formulas	approved	✔	✔
Kal® SAMe 200 mg, 1 Daily, Clear Quality™, Stabilized Active (200 mg/tablet, 1–3/day) Daily: 200–600 mg SAMe enteric coated Mf: Nutraceutical Corp.	approved	✔	✔

Product (label info.)	Test Results		
	Approval	Contained claimed	Broke apart
Life Extension SAMe S-Adenosyl-Methionine 400 mg (400 mg SAMe/ tablet, 2–3/day) Daily: 800–1,200 mg SAMe Dist: Life Extension Foundation	approved	✔	✔
Natrol™ SAMe 200 mg (200 mg/tablet, 2/day) Daily: 400 mg SAMe Dist: Natrol, Inc	approved	✔	✔
Nature Made® Health Solutions® Mood Plus® Improves Mood Naturally SAM-e (200 mg/tablet, 2/day)* Daily: 400 mg SAMe enteric-coated Dist: Nature Made Nutritional Products	approved	✔	✔
Nutralife™ Health Products Incorporated The Original SAMe™, 200 mg active S-adenosyl-methionine per tablet (200 mg/tablet, 2/day) Daily: 400 mg SAMe enteric-coated Dist: NutraLife Health Products Inc.	approved	✔	✔

continued

Product Reviews: Special Ingredients

Product (label info.)	Test Results		
	Approval	Contained claimed	Broke apart
Olympian Labs SAMe Gold 400 mg, Pharmaceutical Grade (400 mg SAMe/tablet, 1–2/day) Daily: 400–800 mg SAMe enteric-coated Dist: Olympian Labs Inc	approved	✔	✔
Vitaline® Formulas (200 mg/tablet, 1–6/day) Daily: 200–1,200 mg SAMe enteric-coated Dist: Integrative Therapeutics Inc	approved	✔	✔
Vitamin Depot® Double Strength SAM-e (S-adenosylmethionine) 400 mg (400 mg/tablet, 1/day)* Daily: 400 mg SAMe enteric-coated Dist: Vitamin Depot	approved	✔	✔

Similar to Approved Product**

Nature's Bounty® SAM-e 400 mg, Double Strength, Enteric Coated and Stomach Friendly (400 mg/tablet, 1–3/day)

Dist: Nature's Bounty, Inc.

‡ See also "More Brand Information," page 675.

✔ Check indicates the results met the criteria listed in the column headings.

*Tested through CL's Voluntary Certification Program prior to, at time of, or after the posting of this Product Review.

**Product identical in formulation and manufacture to a product that has passed testing but sold under a different brand. For more information on CL's Multi-Label Testing Program see Selection and Testing section, page 25, volume 1.

Part 6

Product Reviews: Nutrition Bars, Powders, and Drinks

Nutrition Bars: High-Protein, Low-Carb-Diet, Energy, and Meal-Replacement

Nutrition bars go by many names including "high-protein bars," "low carb/diet bars," "energy bars," and "meal-replacement bars." Nutrition bars are generally much larger by weight than snack bars (such as granola bars) or candy bars (such as chocolate bars) and have a much higher protein content—generally 10 grams to 30 grams of protein in a nutrition bar versus little or no protein in a snack bar or candy bar. (See ConsumerTips™ for Buying and Using, page 551).

Quality Concerns and Product Testing

A concern among bar products, however, is whether they contain what is stated on their labels. In 2001, testing by ConsumerLab.com found most bars to be mislabeled, with many containing undeclared carbohydrates. At around the same time, the U.S. Food and Drug Administration (FDA) sent warning letters to several manufacturers who failed to include certain ingredients in the carbohydrate counts stated on their products. Some labeling discrepancies can be spotted by calculating the expected calories in a product, based on the protein, fat, and carbohydrate contents on the label, and seeing if the total matches the declared calories (see ConsumerTips™ for Buying and Using, page 551). However, most problems, and the magnitude of such problems, can be determined only with laboratory testing.

Neither the FDA, nor any other federal or state agency, routinely tests nutrition bars for quality prior to sale. ConsumerLab.com, as part of its mission to independently evaluate products that affect health, wellness, and nutrition, recently purchased samples of many of the nutrition bars sold in the U.S. (including those designed for diet, energy, protein, or meal replacement) and tested their nutritional claims. The products were analyzed to determine their total calories, total carbohydrates, total sugars, sugar alcohols, total protein, total fat (including a breakout of saturated fat), sodium, and cholesterol. Results were evaluated to determine if the products' labeling claims were accurate (see the appropriate section in "ConsumerLab.com's Testing Methods and Standards," page 669, for more information).

Test Findings

The majority of bars tested met their claims, but the following problems were found in three products:

Detour™ New Triple Layer Deluxe Whey Protein Energy Bar (Caramel Peanut) contained 33% more carbohydrates (8.3 grams) than its stated 25 grams. Keto Bar® (Lemon Chiffon) contained 50% more (1 gram) of saturated fat than its stated 2 grams. Zone Perfect® All Natural Nutrition Bar (Fudge Graham) contained approximately 27% more saturated fat (.8 grams) than the 3 grams claimed.

Differences in the nutritional design among products were striking. Although bars can be a good occasional source of nutrition for people on the go, it is essential that consumers appreciate how one bar may differ from the next and which is best for them. Some of the key differences found among the bars include the following:

"Net Carbs" and Sugar Alcohols: For "low-carb" dieters, many bars displayed a "net carb" calculation that excluded carbohydrates thought to have less impact on blood sugar and insulin levels. This practice has been neither sanctioned nor stopped by the FDA (which also has not authorized the term "low-carb" in labeling). Total carbohydrates in such products often exceed twenty grams per bar, even though the "net carbs" displayed are often only two or three grams. The carbs not counted, typically glycerin and sugar alcohols, still add calories and can easily account for one-quarter of the bar's weight. Some sugar alcohols, such as lactitol, can also have a laxative effect or cause gas.

Bad Fats: At least half the fat in most bars was saturated fat. Saturated fat is associated with an increased risk for heart disease and the USDA recommends that less than 10% of total daily calories should come from saturated fat, which means that less than one-third of total dietary fat should be saturated. As a reference, a product claiming to be "low in saturated fat" must have less than one gram of saturated fat per serving. Amounts of trans fats, also considered bad for the heart, were generally not labeled. These fats can be spotted, however, by looking for "hydrogenated" oils.

Added Vitamins: Many bars were vitamin-fortified. If you take other vitamins or fortified products (such fortified breakfast cereals or vitamin waters), be careful not to exceed tolerable levels. For example, over 10,000 IU of vitamin A (as retinol) daily can weaken bones. And don't give highly fortified bars to young children; the tolerable level of vitamin A for a 3-year-old, for example, is only

2,000 IU per day; a bar with 50% of the adult daily value (DV) contains 1,500 IU. (See "Multivitamin/Multimineral Supplements," page 380.)

Bar as a Meal: If you're replacing a meal with a bar, be sure it contains enough energy. Calories ranged from as much as 330 calories per serving down to only 110 calories, depending on bar size and ingredients. Adults need 2,000 to 3,000 calories a day. If a large amount of a low or no calorie sweetener like sucralose (Splenda) is used, even large bars may leave you hungry. And be sure you get enough protein, which ranged from 3 to 35 grams among the bars studied. You need at least 50 grams of protein a day.

All of the products reviewed were within an acceptable range of their cholesterol and sodium claims, which were generally small amounts. (See ConsumerTips™ for Buying and Using below.)

Test Findings

The 19 products that were selected for testing and a summary of the results are listed alphabetically in Test Results for High-Protein Nutrition Bars, Test Results for Low-Carb/Diet Nutrition Bars, Test Results for Energy Nutrition Bars, and Test Results for Meal-Replacement Bars. Also included in the list are 15 other products (indicated with an asterisk) that have met the same criteria through CL's Voluntary Certification Program (see Selection and Testing, page 25, volume 1). Also shown are the declared weights of the bars, calories, carbohydrates, sugars, protein, total fat and saturated fat, sodium and cholesterol—all of which were checked in testing. In addition, "net carb" statements and trans fats ingredients are provided.

ConsumerTips™ for Buying and Using

Types of Bars: A typical nutrition bar weighs about 60 grams and contains 25 grams of carbohydrates (half from starch and half from sugar), 15 grams of protein, and about 5 grams of fat (of which 3 grams are saturated). About one-quarter of the weight generally comes from water. This typical bar provides 205 calories, with approximately 49% from carbohydrates, 29% from protein, and 22% from fat (13% from saturated fat).

Although definitions are not well established, "energy bars" tend to claim to contain more carbohydrates, "low-carb" and "diet bars" (also called "weight-loss" bars) generally claim to contain fewer carbohydrates (or at least on a "net carb" basis). "High-protein bars" are simply higher in protein and "meal-replacement bars" have more of a balance of carbohydrates, proteins, and fats. Some bars are combinations (such as "meal-replacement, high-protein bars"); others do not claim any specific purpose. Bars may also include vitamins and minerals or other ingredients permitted only in dietary supplements and therefore must be labeled as supplements, rather than foods. Consumers should read labels carefully before using nutrition bars or offering them to children.

How Much Nutrition: The United States Department of Agriculture (USDA) recommends that most adults who perform light to moderate activity get roughly 2,000 to 3,000 calories a day from a varied diet in which about 60% or fewer calories come from carbohydrates, at least 10% come from protein (meats and vegetable proteins), and about 30% come from fats, with less than 10% of calories coming specifically from saturated fat. Healthcare professionals tend to suggest a somewhat higher percentage of calories from protein (15% to 20%) and a lower percentage from carbohydrates, although recommendations vary. Nutrition bars can help provide some of these nutrients, but they are not recommended as a total substitute for food. One downside to many nutrition bars is that they tend to be relatively high in saturated fat, as noted. On the other hand, most bars claim to be low in salt and cholesterol, with a typical bar containing about 150 mg of sodium and generally fewer than 10 mg of cholesterol. The USDA recommends a maximum of 2,400 mg of sodium and 300 mg of cholesterol a day based on a 2,000-calorie diet for a healthy individual.

Serving Sizes: Because some products may contain two or more small bars inside one wrapper, carefully check the "servings per package" information on the label when you are looking for calories and other nutritional figures. Bars can range significantly in terms of calories, protein, carbohydrates, and fats.

To determine if a bar is labeled properly, consider doing the following calculation: multiply the listed weight of each component by the number of calories per gram shown below, and add them together for the total calories.

For example, a product labeled as containing 25 grams of carbohydrates, 15 grams of protein, and 5 grams of fat would have 100 calories from carbohydrates (25 x 4), 60 calories from protein (15 x 4), and 45 calories from fat (5 x 9), for a total of 205 calories.

Calories per Gram	
Carbohydrate (excluding dietary fiber)	4 calories per gram
Protein	4 calories per gram
Fats	9 calories per gram

Carbohydrates would, therefore, contribute about 49% of the calories, protein, about 29%, and fat, about 22%.

If your total is more than a few calories different from what the product label states, the product may be hiding something. (Note that manufacturers are allowed to round off figures and may apply special caloric values to certain ingredients such as sugar and fat substitutes, so don't expect the calculated calories to match the label exactly; allow leeway of up to 10% of the total calories).

Sugar Alcohols and Sugar Substitutes: Although technically carbohydrates, sugar alcohols (also known as polyols) are common in "low-carb" bars because they have fewer calories and less impact than sugar on blood sugar and insulin levels—key elements of low-carb dieting. (Also, because they are digested differently from sugar, they do not promote dental cavities.) Among the most common sugar alcohols in bars are maltitol and lactitol. Unlike sugars, both are primarily digested in the large intestine and consequently may promote gas or have a laxative effect in some people. Unfortunately, most bars don't tell you exactly how much sugar alcohol they contain. If the wrapper of a bar states that "net carbs" are only 2 grams but the Nutrition Facts panel shows 20 grams of carbohydrates, then the bar contains 18 grams of sugar alcohols, glycerin, or fiber. You can also check the ingredient list for sugar alcohols—the higher up in the list, the higher the amount of that ingredient.

Unexpected Ingredients: Some products contain ingredients that you would not expect in a food. A tip-off is if the product states that it is a "Dietary Supplement" or provides a Supplement Facts panel instead of a Nutrition Facts panel. Although this addition is not necessarily a bad thing, just make sure that you are aware of the vitamins, minerals, herbs or other special ingredients that have been added.

You should also be aware that bars, particularly those for energy, might include ingredients containing caffeine such as coffee extract, guarana, green tea or, at lower levels, even cocoa and chocolate. Be aware, too, that caffeine can enhance the action and increase the side effects of other stimulants, such as bitter orange *(Citrus aurantium)*.

As noted, many bars are also fortified with an array of vitamins and minerals. Recommended Tolerable Upper Intake Levels (UL) have been established for many of these vitamins and minerals, so keep track of the amounts that you may be ingesting from the bars as well as from other foods and supplements (see "Multivitamin/ Multimineral Supplements," page 380). Because of all the possible ingredients, nutrition bars should be carefully evaluated before being used by children, pregnant or nursing women, or others with dietary restrictions, such as people with diabetes or hypoglycemia.

Test Results:

High-Protein Nutrition Bars
Low-Carb/Diet Nutrition Bars
Energy Nutrition Bars
Meal-Replacement Bars

Test Results for High-Protein Nutrition Bars

Product (flavor)/bar size‡ Test results Manufacturer (Mf) or distributor (Dist)	Nutrition or supplement facts on label (Per bar unless otherwise noted)			
	Calories	Total carb (g)	Sugars (g)	Net carb claim
Detour™ New Triple Layer Deluxe Whey Protein Energy Bar (Caramel Peanut)/80 g **_not_ approved (Contained 33.3 grams of carbohydrates. Claimed only 25)** Dist: Next Proteins™	310	25	12	N/A
GeniSoy® Delicious Soy Protein Bar (Ultimate Chocolate Fudge Brownie)/61.5 g **✔—Passed Testing** GeniSoy Products Co.	240	35	22	N/A
Kashi® GoLean® High Protein & Fiber Bar (Peanut Butter & Chocolate)/78 g **✔—Passed Testing** Dist: Kashi Company	290	48	31	N/A
Met-Rx® Sports Nutrition Protein Plus® Protein Bar (Chocolate Roasted Peanut)/85 g* **✔—Passed Testing** Dist: Met-Rx USA Inc.	330	32	10	N/A

	Protein (g)	Total fat (g)	Sat. fat (g)	Trans fat	Sodium (mg)	Cholesterol (mg)
	30	10	4	Partially hydroge-nated palm kernel oil	480	40
	14	5	3	None listed	210	0
	13	6	4.5	None listed	280	0
	32	9	4.5	None listed	350	10

continued

Product (flavor)/bar size‡ Test results	Nutrition or supplement facts on label			
	Calories	Total carb (g)	Sugars (g)	Net carb claim
Nutrilite® Trim Advantage® Protein Bar (Fudgy Brownie with Almonds)/ 60 g* ✔—Passed Testing Dist: Access Business Group International LLC	260	25	10	Net Carb Count: 3 grams. Maltitol, sucralose, glycerine and fiber not included.
Muscletech Delicious High-Protein Bar Nitro-Tech™ (Chocolate Peanut Butter Delight)/88 g ✔—Passed Testing Dist: MuscleTech R & D, Inc.	290	31	2	Net Carb Count: 3 grams. Lactitol, maltitol, and fiber not included.
Promax™ Great Tasting Energy Bar (Cookies 'n Cream)/75 g ✔—Passed Testing Dist: Promax Nutrition Inc.	290	38	25	N/A
Pure Protein® Protein Revolution® High Protein Triple Layer Bar (Chocolate Peanut Caramel)/78 g* ✔—Passed Testing Dist: Worldwide Sport Nutritional Supplements, Inc.	280	26	2	Net Carb Count: 3 grams. Maltitol, sucralose, glycerin, and fiber not included.

N/A—Not applicable.
‡ See also "More Brand Information," page 675.
*Tested through CL's Voluntary Certification Program before, at the time of, or after the initial review

Protein (g)	Total fat (g)	Sat. fat (g)	Trans fat	Sodium (mg)	Cholesterol (mg)
22	10	1	0	230	10
35	7	4.5	partially hydroge-nated palm oil	230	<5
20	6	3	0 g; partially hydro-genated soybean and/or cottonseed oil	200	5
32	9	6	0	240	15

Test Results for Low-Carb/Diet Nutrition Bars

Product (flavor)/bar size‡ Test results Manufacturer (Mf) or distributor (Dist)	Nutrition or supplement facts on label (Per bar unless otherwise noted)			
	Calories	Total carb (g)	Sugars (g)	Net carb claim
Atkins™ Advantage™ (Chocolate Peanut Butter Bar)/60 g ✔—**Passed Testing** Dist: Atkins Nutritionals, Inc.	240	21	1	Net carb count: 2 grams. Sucralose, glycerin, and fiber not included.
Carb Minders™ High Protein Bar for Low-Carb Diets (Crispy Chocolate Peanut Bars)/60 g* ✔—**Passed Testing** Dist: HealthSmart	240	23	1	Net carb count: 3 grams. Maltitol, lactitol, sucralose, glycerin, and fiber not included.
Carb Minders™ High Protein Bar for Low-Carb Diets, (Crispy Chocolate S'mores Bars)/60 g* ✔—**Passed Testing** Dist: HealthSmart	240	23	1	Net carb count: 2 grams. Maltitol, lactitol, sucralose, glycerin, and fiber not included.
Carb Minders™ High Protein Bar for Low-Carb Diets (Crispy Lemon Yogurt Bars)/60 g* ✔—**Passed Testing** Dist: HealthSmart	240	23	1	Net carb count: 4 grams. Maltitol, lactitol, sucralose, glycerine, and fiber not included.

Protein (g)	Total fat (g)	Sat. fat (g)	Trans fat	Sodium (mg)	Cholesterol (mg)
19	12	6	None listed	180	<5
21	10	5	None listed	320	0
20	9	6	None listed	330	0
20	9	6	None listed	320	0

continued

Product (flavor)/bar size‡ Test results	Nutrition or supplement facts on label			
	Calories	Total carb (g)	Sugars (g)	Net carb claim
Carb Minders™ High Protein Bar for Low-Carb Diets (Crispy Raspberry Bars)/60 g* ✔—Passed Testing Dist: HealthSmart	240	24	2	Net carb count: 3 grams. Maltitol, lactitol, sucralose, glycerin, and fiber not included.
Carb Options™ (Chocolate Chip Brownie Bar)/50 g ✔—Passed Testing Dist: Unilever Bestfoods	200	17	0	Net Carb Count: 2 grams. Maltitol, erythritol, sucralose, glycerin, and fiber not included.
Carb Solutions™ Good Mornings!™ Breakfast & Lunch Bars (Pecan Cinnamon Bun)/37 g* ✔—Passed Testing Dist: Richardson Labs, Inc.	150	14	1	Net Carb Count: 2 grams. Maltitol, sucralose, glycerin, and fiber not included.
Carb Solutions™ High Protein Bar for Low Carb Diets, Taste Sensations!™ (Creamy Chocolate Peanut Butter)/60 g* ✔—Passed Testing Dist: Richardson Labs, Inc.	250	14	1	Net carb count: 3 grams. Maltitol, sucralose, glycerin, and fiber not included.

	Protein (g)	Total fat (g)	Sat. fat (g)	Trans fat	Sodium (mg)	Cholesterol (mg)
	21	9	6	None listed	330	0
	16	8	4	0 g; partially hydro-genated vegetable oil (palm kernel, palm), partially hydro-genated palm oil	200	<5
	13	7	3.5	partially hydro-genated palm oil	160	0
	250	12	3.5	None listed	210	<5

continued

Product (flavor)/bar size‡ Test results	Nutrition or supplement facts on label			
	Calories	Total carb (g)	Sugars (g)	Net carb claim
CarboRite™ Sugar Free (Crispy Caramel Bar)/32 g **✔—Passed Testing** Dist: CarboLite™ Foods, Inc.	120	18	0	Net carb count: 0.7 grams. Maltitol, sucralose, and fiber not included.
Delicious Crispy CarbWise™ High Protein Bar for Low-Carb Diets (Chocolate Peanut Crunch)/60 g* **✔—Passed Testing** Dist: CarbWise A Division of Synergy Plus	240	23	1	Net carb count: 3 grams. Maltitol, lactitol, sucralose, glycerin, and fiber not included.
Dexatrim™ All in One Energizing Nutritious Delicious Diet Bar (Chocolate Toffee Crunch)/50 g **✔—Passed Testing** Dist: Chattem, Inc.	180	20	1	Net carb count: 1 grams. Maltitol, sucralose, glycerin, and fiber not included.
Keto Bar® (Lemon Chiffon)/65 g **_not_ approved (Contained 3 grams of saturated fat; claimed only 2.0)** Mf: Keto Foods and Snacks, Inc.	230	21	<1	Net carb count: 2 grams. Maltitol, sucralose, and fiber not included.

	Protein (g)	Total fat (g)	Sat. fat (g)	Trans fat	Sodium (mg)	Cholesterol (mg)
	3	7	4.5	partially hydro-genated soybean oil	25	5
	21	10	5	None listed	320	0
	15	5	3.5	None listed	190	<5
	24	6	2	None listed	180	30

continued

Product (flavor)/bar size‡ Test results	Nutrition or supplement facts on label			
	Calories	Total carb (g)	Sugars (g)	Net carb claim
PowerBar® Pria™ CarbSelect™ (Peanut Butter Caramel Nut)/48 g* ✔—Passed Testing Dist: PowerBar, Inc.	170	21	1	Net carb count: 2 grams. Sucralose, glycerin, and fiber not included.
Rich & Creamy CarbWise™ Gold High Protein Bar for Low-Carb Diets (Chocolate Caramel Peanut)/50 g* ✔—Passed Testing Dist: CarbWise, a Division of Synergy Plus	190	18	1	Net Carb Count: 3 grams. Maltitol, lactitol, sucralose, glycerin, and fiber not included.
Think Thin! Low Carb Diet (Chocolate Fudge)/60 g ✔—Passed Testing Dist: Prime Health Dietary Supplements, Inc.	230	23	0	Net carb count: 2 grams. Maltitol, glycerin, and fiber not included.

‡ See also "More Brand Information," page 675.

*Tested through CL's Voluntary Certification Program before, at the time of, or after the initial review.

Protein (g)	Total fat (g)	Sat. fat (g)	Trans fat	Sodium (mg)	Cholesterol (mg)
10	8	5	0	160	5
18	7	4	partially hydro-genated soybean oil	160	<5
20	7	3.5	None listed	150	5

Test Results for Energy Nutrition Bars

Product (flavor)/bar size‡ Test results Manufacturer (Mf) or distributor (Dist)	Nutrition or supplement facts on label (Per bar unless otherwise noted)			
	Calories	Total carb (g)	Sugars (g)	Net carb claim
151 Energy Bar, Fresh Baked Taste (Fruit Burst)/63 g ✔—Passed Testing (Contained 6.5 g/sugar alcohol**) Dist: Applied Nutrition®	230	46	25	N/A
Balance® High Protein, 40-30-30 Nutrition, Complete Nutrition Energy Bar (Yogurt Honey Peanut Natural Flavor)/50 g ✔—Passed Testing Dist: Balance Bar Company	200	22	18	N/A
Clif Luna®, The Whole Nutrition Bar for Women, (Lemon-zest®)/48 g ✔—Passed Testing Dist: Clif Bar Inc.	180	26	14	N/A
EAS™ Myoplex® Lite (Cinnamon Roll Crisp)/54 g ✔—Passed Testing Dist: EAS, Inc.	190	27	16	N/A

Protein (g)	Total fat (g)	Sat. fat (g)	Trans fat	Sodium (mg)	Cholesterol (mg)
3	4	0	None listed	50	0
15	6	3	None listed	160	<5
10	4	3	None listed	50	0
15	4.5	2.5	None listed	280	<5

continued

| Product (flavor)/bar size‡ | Nutrition or supplement facts on label | | | |
	Calories	Total carb (g)	Sugars (g)	Net carb claim
PowerBar® Pria™ Deliciously Smarter™ Nutritional Energy Snack Bar (Mint Chocolate Cookie)/28 g* ✔—Passed Testing Dist: PowerBar, Inc.	110	16	9	N/A
PowerBar® The Original Performance Energy Bar™ (Cookies & Cream)/65 g* ✔—Passed Testing Dist: PowerBar, Inc.	240	45	20	N/A
Snickers® Marathon™ Long Lasting Energy Bar (Multi-Grain Crunch with Quadratein™ Protein Blend)/55 g ✔—Passed Testing Dist: Master-foods USA	220	32	18	N/A
XS™ Power Nutrition Energy Bars (Caramel Peanut)/46 g* ✔—Passed Testing Dist: Access Business Group International LLC	180	18	6	N/A

	Protein (g)	Total fat (g)	Sat. fat (g)	Trans fat	Sodium (mg)	Cholesterol (mg)
	5	3.5	2.5	None listed	90	<5
	9	3.5	0.5	None listed	120	<5
	9	7	2	partially hydroge-nated soy-bean oil	210	5
	15	6	2.5	partially hydroge-nated soy-bean and cottonseed oil	170	0

continued

Product Reviews: Nutrition Bars, Powders, and Drinks

Product (flavor)/bar size‡ Test results	Nutrition or supplement facts on label			
	Calories	Total carb (g)	Sugars (g)	Net carb claim
Zone Perfect® All Natural Nutrition Bar (Fudge Graham)/50 g **not approved (Contained 3.8 grams of saturated fat; claimed only 3)** Dist: ZonePerfect Nutrition Company	210	22	13	N/A

N/A—Not applicable.
‡ See also "More Brand Information," page 675.
*Tested through CL's Voluntary Certification Program before, at the time of, or after the initial review.
**The sugar alcohol found in this product may be natural occurring from fruits listed as ingredients. Daily consumption of three bars, however, may provide sufficient sugar alcohol to cause a laxative effect.

Protein (g)	Total fat (g)	Sat. fat (g)	Trans fat	Sodium (mg)	Cholesterol (mg)
16	7	3	None listed	250	0

Test Results for Meal-Replacement Nutrition Bars

Product (flavor)/bar size‡ Test results Manufacturer (Mf) or distributor (Dist)	Nutrition or supplement facts on label (Per bar unless otherwise noted)			
	Calories	Total carb (g)	Sugars (g)	Net carb claim
Dr. Sears™ Patented Zone Meal with EPA & DHA, Omega-Zone™ Controlled Release Nutrition (Chocolate)/55 g ✔ — Passed Testing Dist: Sears Labs, Inc.	210	25	17	N/A
Nutrilite® Trim Advantage® Meal Replacement Bar (Chocolate Flavor with Coconut)/60 g* ✔ — Passed Testing Dist: Access Business Group International LLC	230	26	16	N/A
Slim-Fast® Meal Options® Breakfast & Lunch Bars (Dutch Chocolate)/34 g ✔ — Passed Testing Dist: Slim-Fast Foods Company	140	20	12	N/A

N/A—Not applicable.
‡ See also "More Brand Information," page 675.
*Tested through CL's Voluntary Certification Program before, at the time of, or after the initial review.

Protein (g)	Total fat (g)	Sat. fat (g)	Trans fat	Sodium (mg)	Cholesterol (mg)
15	6	2.5	None listed	150	15
15	8	6	None listed	220	0
5	5	3	0; partially hydrogenated vegetable oil	85	5

Nutrition Powders, Shakes and Drinks: Protein, Diet, General Nutrition, and Meal-Replacements

What sets nutrition powders and drinks apart from most other beverages is their high protein content (ranging from about 10 to 50 grams a serving) as well as added vitamins, minerals, or other dietary supplement ingredients. The powders typically come in canisters or packets ready to be mixed with water, milk, juice, or other beverage. Drinks commonly come in ready-to-use cans. These products are marketed as dieting aids, meal replacements, energy boosters, and concentrated sources of protein.

Although nutrition bars need to contain at least 15 grams of carbohydrate to give them a reasonable texture, feel, and taste, nutrition powders and drinks do not (see "Nutrition Bars: High-Protein, Low-Carb-Diet, Energy, and Meal-Replacement," page 549). Consequently, makers of nutrition powders and drinks have a great deal of flexibility in the nutritional content of these products. For example, it is quite possible to find powders and drinks with half the fat and carbohydrates of most nutrition bars, though they commonly offer twice the protein. Of course, with powders, these nutritional numbers can change significantly depending on the liquid used with the mix (see ConsumerTips™ for Buying and Using, page 579). In general, drinks and powders tend to have slightly fewer calories per serving than bars, but again, this may not be the case if a powder is mixed with a high-calorie liquid, such as whole milk.

The United States Department of Agriculture (USDA) recommends that most adults who perform light to moderate activity get roughly 2,000 to 3,000 calories per day from a varied diet in which roughly 60% or fewer calories come from carbohydrates, at least 10% come from protein (meats and vegetable proteins), and about 30% come from fats, with less than 10% of calories coming specifically from saturated fat. Healthcare professionals tend to suggest a somewhat higher percentage of calories from protein (15% to 20%) and a lower percentage from carbohydrates, although recommendations vary.

Nutrition powders and drinks can provide some of these nutrients, but they are not a total substitute for food because they lack some of the vitamins, minerals, fiber, and phytonutrients found in whole foods and sometimes fall short on fat and carbohydrates.

The average serving of a powder is about 45 grams (about the same as that for a nutrition bar, after taking into account the bar's moisture content), although recommended serving sizes vary widely among the powders (from as little as 10 grams to more than 80 grams). As an example, in a 45-gram serving of a high-protein powdered mix, you could expect about 10 grams of carbohydrate (of which sugar may account for two-thirds, unless a non-nutritive sweetener is used), 30 grams of protein, and 2 grams of fat (a third of which is saturated). The other few grams of weight come mostly from moisture. This powder would provide 178 calories, with approximately 23% from carbohydrates, 67% from protein, and 10% from fat. (See ConsumerTips™ for Buying and Using, page 579, for calculating calories and information about the forms of protein—whey, casein, and soy.) Therefore, powders can be a great source of protein, but can leave you short on carbohydrates and fat, if mixed with water. A typical serving of a ready-to-use nutrition drink is about 315 mL (1⅓ cups). Nutrients in a drink can be similar to that for a powder, but typically have slightly less protein and slightly more carbohydrate and fat.

Quality Concerns and Product Testing

Neither the U.S. Food and Drug Administration (FDA), nor any other federal or state agency, routinely tests nutrition powders and drinks for quality prior to sale. Some labeling discrepancies can be spotted by calculating the expected calories in a product, based on the protein, fat, and carbohydrate contents on the label, and determining if the total calories match the calories actually listed on the label. However, most problems, and the magnitude of such problems, can be determined only with laboratory testing.

To determine if such problems might exist with nutrition powders and drinks, and as part of its mission to independently evaluate products that affect health, wellness, and nutrition, ConsumerLab.com purchased a variety of nutrition powders and drinks. The products were first evaluated to make sure that their listed ingredients and claims were in compliance with FDA labeling regulations. Products were then tested for the accuracy of their label claims regarding total calories, total carbohydrates, total sugars, total protein, total fat (including a breakout of saturated fat), sodium, and cholesterol (see "ConsumerLab.com's Testing Methods and Standards," page 669).

Test Findings

The majority of products tested met their claims, but three products contained more sodium than claimed and two contained more cholesterol. The extra amounts are not terribly high, but should be of concern to anyone trying to restrict their intake of sodium and cholesterol.

Products with more sodium than claimed: GeniSoy® Soy Protein Powder, Fat Free, No Cholesterol contained 423 mg of sodium, 51% more than its stated 280 mg per serving. ISS Complete Whey Power™, 99% Pure Whey Protein, Cookies & Cream did not list any sodium on its label, but tested to contain 35 mg per serving. Now® Eco-Green Protein Powder, Non-GE Soy Protein, Vanilla Drink Mix contained 229 mg of sodium, 43% more than its stated 160 mg per serving.

To put these sodium amounts into perspective, the amount of sodium in one "shake" of salt is about 15 mg (depending on the shaker, of course). For a product to be considered "low in sodium," it must contain less than 140 mg of sodium. For a healthy adult under age fifty, total daily intake of sodium should be about 1,500 mg (1,300 mg for those age 50 to 70 and 1,200 mg for those age 71 and older) and should not exceed 2,300 mg. Be aware, however, that a study found that more than 95% of men and 75% of women exceed these upper levels, which may contribute to high blood pressure. In addition, more restricted sodium intake applies to people who are particularly sensitive to the blood pressure effects of sodium: older persons, African Americans, and individuals with hypertension, diabetes, or chronic kidney disease. However, individuals who are active in hot environments and are losing sodium from sweat may need more sodium.

Products with more cholesterol than claimed include the following: Designer Whey™ Protein, 2g net sugar carbs, French Vanilla Protein Supplement, New & Improved, contained 48 mg of cholesterol, 60% more than its stated 30 mg per serving.

ON's Instantized 100% Whey Protein Dietary Supplement, Double Rich Chocolate contained 19 mg of cholesterol, nearly double its stated 10 mg per serving. Most recommendations are that a healthy adult consume no more than 300 mg of cholesterol per day.

The 16 products that were selected for testing and a summary of the results are listed alphabetically in Test Results for Nutrition Powders, Shakes, and Drinks. Also included in the list are 21 other products (indicated with an asterisk) that have met the same criteria through CL's Voluntary Certification Program (see Selection and Testing, page 25, volume 1). NOTE: Products are grouped by type of use and appear alphabetically within these groups. Some products could be categorized into more than one group, e.g., "Diet/Meal Replacement" and "Protein," but are shown in one category only.

ConsumerTips™ for Buying and Using

Serving Sizes: Suggested serving sizes vary widely among powders and drinks, ranging from 10 grams to more than 80 grams a serving among powders and from one cup (237 mL or 8 fluid ounces) to almost three cups for drinks. Keep this variation in mind when comparing the nutritional quality of products as well as cost.

Protein: The American Dietetic Association (ADA) currently recognizes a daily protein requirement of about 0.40 gram/pound of body weight for sedentary individuals, 0.55 to 0.65 gram/pound for endurance athletes, and 0.65 to 0.80 gram/pound for strength-training athletes. The ADA also states that the maximum usable protein for adults is 1 gram/pound. To get more protein in the diet, you can turn to meats, but these may also add saturated fats and cholesterol to your diet. Another alternative is to combine large servings of incomplete proteins such as legumes and grains, but this increases carbohydrate and calorie intake. Powders and drinks offer a protein alternative without significantly increasing consumption of fats, carbohydrates, cholesterol, or calories.

Increased protein in the diet results in increased protein metabolism and urea production, which in turn increases urine output. The combined factors of a high protein intake and an inadequate fluid intake can result in severe dehydration. Overall, remember to increase fluid consumption if your diet requires a higher than normal amount of protein. High-protein diets can also increase calcium turnover from bone, resulting in calcium loss. However, this can be stabilized by the daily consumption of 300 mg of calcium (the equivalent to one 8 oz. glass of milk).

Three types of protein—whey, casein, and soy—are commonly found in nutrition powders and drinks. Whey and casein are both derived from milk (the protein in milk is 80% casein and 20% whey). Soy is vegetable-based. However, keep in mind that many products are made from a mixture of protein sources and the relative amounts of each type are generally not well revealed.

Whey protein: The majority of "protein" products on the market are whey-based. Because it is milk-derived, powders and drinks made with whey are likely to have some milk fats (about 1 to 2 grams per serving) and a small amount of cholesterol (about 25 milligrams [mg] per serving). The USDA recommends a maximum of 300 mg of cholesterol per day based on a 2,000-calorie diet for a healthy individual, so the cholesterol from whey protein is minimal.

Whey is a "complete" protein, meaning that it contains all the essential amino acids and contains the highest branched chain amino acid (BCAA) content found in nature. The branched chain amino acids valine, leucine, and isoleucine tend to become depleted following exercise and are needed for the maintenance of muscle tissue. Whey protein is thought to be digested faster than casein and more completely than soy protein. Some human and animal studies have also suggested it may boost the body's ability to fight cancer.

Popular forms of whey include the following: whey hydrosolates, whey isolates, and ion-exchange purified whey. Whey hydrosolates are essentially predigested protein that is assimilated into the body more quickly than other, nonhydrolyzed types. This quick assimilation is well suited for use after exercise because of the increased bioavailability of the predigested protein. Also, because these products are predigested, less energy is needed to digest them. Whey isolates are purified without the use of heat. Thus, they still contain the potentially beneficial immunostimulant constituents (immunoglobulins) of whey. Whey protein "isolates" are typically lower in lactose, fat, and cholesterol than regular whey protein. Ion-exchange purified whey is the most pure of all the whey proteins, but may have reduced immunostimulant properties due to chemical processing. All whey proteins should be avoided by anyone who is allergic to milk proteins.

Casein: The other milk protein, casein, is also a "complete protein" and is extremely high in glutamine, the predominant amino acid in your muscles and body. However, casein has a lower biological value (BV) than whey, meaning that a lower percentage of protein is absorbed from the total protein consumed. Casein is larger than whey, and is not as bioavailable. Studies have shown casein to lead to superior gains in strength over whey, most likely because of the slower absorption of casein, providing a release of amino acids over a longer period. For athletes looking to maintain lean muscle tissue, casein may be more beneficial before bed because the slow absorption will supply the body with protein through the night when the body enters a catabolic state (breakdown of protein tissue for

580

energy). Popular forms of casein are micellar casein (the natural, undenatured form of casein found in milk) and calcium caseinate, which is a good source of calcium.

Soy: Soy is the most "heart healthy" source of protein, as well as being acceptable to vegetarians. Research clearly shows that soy can lower cholesterol levels. In addition, according to the FDA, eating 25 grams of soy protein a day, in addition to eating a low-fat, low-cholesterol diet, can reduce your risk of heart disease. Soy does not contain much fat or cholesterol, particularly if a soy "isolate" is used. Soy isolates may also provide higher amounts of soy isoflavones such as genistein, daidzein, and glycitein than a soy protein concentrate, offering other benefits such as a reduction in menopausal symptoms (see "Menopausal Symptom-Relief Supplements: Soy and Red Clover Isoflavones, Black Cohosh, and Progesterone Cream," page 116, volume 1, for more information about isoflavones).

However, soy protein is not a complete protein because it lacks the sulfur-containing amino acid methionine. And the processing to produce the soy protein isolates can cause the loss of cysteine and lysine. These sulfur-containing amino acids are particularly important for protein synthesis, growth, and proper immune system function.

Anyone with thyroid disease or a predisposition to thyroid dysfunction should limit his or her intake of soy-based protein food because of its potential to affect hormone balance. Although soy allergies are rare, anyone allergic to soybeans should also avoid soy protein.

Unexpected Ingredients: Some products contain ingredients that you would not expect in a food. It helps to look closely at the label to see if the product claims to be a "Dietary Supplement," because such a label may indicate that it contains nonfood ingredients, although it is also required if a product is making a claim of how it can help support certain body functioning or structure. Although such supplementation is not necessarily a bad thing, you should be aware of the vitamins, minerals, herbs, or other special ingredients that have been added. Recommended Tolerable Upper Intake Levels (UL) have been established for many vitamins and minerals, so it is advisable to keep track of the amounts that you may be ingesting from the powders and drinks as well as from other foods and supplements. See ConsumerTips™ for Buying and Using in "Multivitamin/Multimineral Supplements," page 384, for Recommended Dietary Allowances (RDA) and (UL).

You should also be aware that "energy" products may include caffeine-containing ingredients, such as coffee extract, guarana, maté, or cocoa. Caffeine can enhance the action and increase the side effects of other stimulants.

Powders and drinks may also contain an array of sweeteners. Some are sugar-based such as sugar, fructose, honey, lactose, maltose, and fruit juices. Some have reduced calories, such as the sugar alcohols lactitol, maltitol, mannitol, sorbitol, and xylitol. And some have no calories, such as saccharin, aspartame, acesulfame-K, and sucralose. In addition, some products now have a "net carb" calculation on their labels. In this calculation, the manufacturer deducts the weight of any carbohydrate (including sugars) that supposedly does not raise insulin levels, although the carbohydrates still contribute calories. The FDA has not approved this practice.

Because of all the possible ingredients, nutritional products should be carefully evaluated before being used by children, pregnant or nursing women, or others with dietary restrictions, such as people with diabetes or hypoglycemia.

Calories Add Up: To make sure that the calories listed on a product match up with the listed nutrients, you may want to do the following calculation: multiply the listed weight of each component by the number of calories per gram as shown in the table, and add them together for the total number of calories.

Calories per Gram	
Carbohydrate (excluding dietary fiber)	4 calories per gram
Protein	4 calories per gram
Fats	9 calories per gram

For example, a product labeled as containing 25 grams of carbohydrates, 15 grams of protein, and 5 grams of fat would have 100 calories from carbohydrates (25 x 4), 60 calories from protein (15 x 4), and 45 calories from fat (5 x 9), for a total of 205 calories. Carbohydrates would, therefore, contribute about 49% of the calories, protein, about 29%, and fat, about 22%.

If your total is more than a few calories off from label statement, the product may be hiding something. NOTE: manufacturers are allowed to round numbers and certain sugar and fat substitutes may have fewer calories than normal sugars and fats, so don't expect the calculated calories to match the label exactly; allow leeway of up to 10% of the total calories.

Nutritional Content of Liquids: The nutritional profile of a drink made from powder obviously depends on the liquid used in the mix. "Nutrients in Common Liquids Mixed with Nutrition Powders" lists the nutritional content of some of the most common liquids used, besides water. Figures shown are based on one cup of liquid (8 fluid ounces), but the suggested amount of liquid per serving varies by product. In general, most powders suggest about one cup of liquid per 40 grams of powder (roughly two medium scoops).

Nutrients in Common Liquids Mixed with Nutrition Powder

Liquid (1 cup)	Calories	Carbohydrate (g)	Fat (g)	Protein (g)
Whole milk	149	11	8	8
Skim milk	86	12	0	8
Orange juice	110	25	1	2
Apple juice	117	29	0	0

Source: U.S. Department of Agriculture, Agricultural Research Service. 2001. USDA Nutrient Database for Standard Reference, Release 14. Nutrient Data Laboratory Home Page,
http://www.nal.usda.gov/fnic/foodcomp.

Test Results for Nutrition Powders, Shakes, and Drinks

Product, flavor, serving size†‡ Manufacturer (Mf) or distributor (Dist)	Approved or not approved	Nutrition or supplement (Figures are per serving)		
		Total fat (g)	Sat. fat (g)	Sodium (mg)
Protein				
Body Fortress® Precision Engineered™ Whey Protein, Pure Whey Protein Powder, Chocolate Flavor, serving size: 23 g (1 scoop)* Mf: U.S. Nutrition	approved	1	0	200
Carb Watchers™ Proplete Gold® Premium Whey Protein, Great for Carb Restricted Diets, Banana Creme Flavor with Real Bits of Bananas, serving size: 31.4 g (1 scoop) Dist: Labrada Nutrition	approved	2	1	45
Designer Whey™ Protein, 2g net sugar carbs, French Vanilla Protein Supplement, New & Improved, serving size: 24 g (1 scoop) Dist: Next Proteins™	**not** approved; extra 18 mg of cholesterol/ serving (60% above label claim)	1.5	0.5	60

584

	Cholesterol (mg)	Total carb	Sugar (g)	Protein (g)	Calories
	20	2	1	17	80
	60	5	3	21	120
	30	2	2	18	90

continued

Product Reviews: Nutrition Bars, Powders, and Drinks

Product flavor, serving size†	Approval	Nutrition or supplement		
		Total fat (g)	Sat. fat (g)	Sodium (mg)
EAS™ Myoplex® Original Advanced Protein, Ready to Drink, New and Improved Formula, Chocolate Fudge, serving size: 500 mL (1 can) Dist: EAS, Inc.	approved	7	1	610
GeniSoy® Soy Protein Powder, Fat Free, No Cholesterol, serving size: 30 g (1 scoop) Dist: GeniSoy Products Co.	**not** approved; additional 143 mg of sodium/ serving (51% above label claim)	0	0	280
GNC Pro Perfomance® 50 Gram Slam™ Protein Drink, Milk Chocolate, serving size: 444 mL (1 can)* Dist: General Nutrition Corporation	approved	2	1	160
GNC Pro-Perfomance® Mega Whey Extreme™, Chocolate, serving size: 82 g (3 scoops)* Dist: General Nutrition Corporation	approved	2	1	450

Cholesterol (mg)	Total carb	Sugar (g)	Protein (g)	Calories
20	20	2	43	310
0	0	0	25	100
40	12	4	50	270
30	13	1	60	310

continued

Product Reviews: Nutrition Bars, Powders, and Drinks

Product flavor, serving size†	Approval	Nutrition or supplement		
		Total fat (g)	Sat. fat (g)	Sodium (mg)
Herbalife® Bulk & Muscle Formula Protein Drink Mix, Vanilla, serving size: 60 g (1 scoop) Dist: Herbalife International of America, Inc.	approved	1	0	310
ISS Complete Whey Power™, 99% Pure Whey Protein, Cookies & Cream, serving size: 22.2 g (1 scoop) Dist: Integrated Sports Science	**not** approved; *35* mg sodium/ serving; none claimed on label	2	0	0
MET-Rx® Engineered Nutrition® Ultramyosyn™ Whey Advanced Protein Powder Fast Acting Protein, Vanilla, serving size: 28.3 g (2 scoops)* Mf: MET-Rx USA, Inc.	approved	2	1.5	80
Muscletech™ Nitro-Tech™, Advanced Musclebuilding Protein Formula™, Delicious Strawberry, Dietary Supplement: serving size: 28.5 g (1 scoop) Dist: MuscleTech R & D, Inc.	approved	1.5	1	60

Cholesterol (mg)	Total carb	Sugar (g)	Protein (g)	Calories
<5	2	13	30	210
40	3	1	17	80
55	3	2	20	110
30	4	2	20	100

continued

Product flavor, serving size†	Approval	Nutrition or supplement		
		Total fat (g)	Sat. fat (g)	Sodium (mg)
Now® Eco-Green Protein Powder, Non-GE Soy Protein, Vanilla Drink Mix, serving size: 34 g (1 scoop) Mf: NOW Foods	*not approved; extra 69 mg of sodium/ serving (43% above label claim)*	1	0	160
Nutrilite XS™ Power Nutrition Protein Shake, Chocolate Fudge, serving size: 325 mL (1 can)* Dist: Access Business Group Intl. LLC	approved	6	1	45
Nutrilite® Protein Powder, serving size: 12.5 g (1 scoop)* Dist: Access Business Group Intl. LLC	approved	<0.5	0	95
ON's Instantized 100% Whey Protein Dietary Supplement, Double Rich Chocolate, serving size: 29.4 g (1 scoop) Mf: ON (Optimum Nutrition)	*not approved; extra 9.4 mg of cholesterol/ serving (94% above label claim)*	1.5	0.5	40
Precision Engineered® Protoplex Deluxe, Deluxe Vanilla Flavor, serving size: 82 g (3 scoops)* Mf: U.S. Nutrition	approved	2	0.5	350

Cholesterol (mg)	Total carb	Sugar (g)	Protein (g)	Calories
0	13	8	16	130
10	6	1	35	220
1	1	0	10	45
10	3	1	23	110
5	27	1	42	290

continued

Product flavor, serving size†	Approval	Nutrition or supplement		
		Total fat (g)	Sat. fat (g)	Sodium (mg)
Precision Engineered® Protoplex Lite, Vanilla Flavor, serving size: 56.8 g (2 scoops)* Mf: U.S. Nutrition	approved	1.5	0	330
Precision Engineered® Protopure, Vanilla Flavor, serving size: 86 g (3 scoops)* Mf: U.S. Nutrition	approved	0.5	0	210
Precision Engineered® Whey Protein Pure Whey Protein Powder, Vanilla Flavor, serving size: 22.2 g (1 scoop)* Mf: U.S. Nutrition	approved	1.5	0	60
Puritan's Pride® Pure Soy Protein Isolate Powder, serving size: 28.4 g (1 scoop)* Mf: Puritan's Pride, Inc.	approved	1	0	250
Puritan's Pride® Vanilla Soy Protein Powder, serving size: 29 g (1 scoop)* Mf: Puritan's Pride, Inc.	approved	1	0	260

Cholesterol (mg)	Total carb	Sugar (g)	Protein (g)	Calories
5	19	1	25	190
0	25	1	50	300
35	1	<1	17	90
0	0	0	25	110
0	<1	0	25	110

continued

Product flavor, serving size†	Approval	Nutrition or supplement		
		Total fat (g)	Sat. fat (g)	Sodium (mg)
Solgar® Whey To Go® Ion-Exchanged, Micro-Filtered and Hydrolyzed Whey Protein Powder, Natural Mixed Berry Flavor, serving size: 28.4 g (1 scoop)* Dist: Solgar Vitamin and Herb	approved	<1	<0.5	75
Vital Nutrients NaturalSoy, Organic Non-Genetically Engineered Fermented Soy Powder, All Vegetarian Formula, serving size: 30 g (3 Tbsp.) Mf: Vital Nutrients	approved	5.8	0.67	12.7
Vitamin World® Value Whey™ Protein Powder, Vanilla Flavor, serving size: 28 g (1 scoop)* Mf: Vitamin World, Inc.	approved	2.5	1.5	60
Vitamin World® Vanilla Soy Protein Isolate Powder, serving size: 29.4 g (1 scoop)* Mf: Vitamin World, Inc.	approved	1	0	250

Cholesterol (mg)	Total carb	Sugar (g)	Protein (g)	Calories
10	8	7	16	100
0	9.4	2.5	11	134
60	3	1	19	110
0	0	0	25	110

continued

Product flavor, serving size†	Approval	Nutrition or supplement		
		Total fat (g)	Sat. fat (g)	Sodium (mg)
Worldwide Sports Nutrition® Extreme Whey Protein Powder, Vanilla, serving size: 29 g (2 scoops)* Mf: Worldwide, Inc.	approved	2	1.5	150
Zone Perfect® Protein Powder Supplement, All Natural Premium Soy & Whey Protein Blend, serving size: 9 g (1 scoop) Dist: ZonePerfect Nutrition Co.	approved	0	0	50
General Nutrition				
Atkins® Advantage™, The Original Low Carb Lifestyle™, Shake Mix, Strawberry, serving size: 33 g (2 scoops) Dist: Atkins Nutritionals, Inc.	approved	4	0	75
Puritan's Pride® Dietary Supplement, Life's Greens® With Advanced Probiotic Formula, serving size: 9 g (1 scoop)* Dist: Puritan's Pride, Inc.	approved	2	0	35

Cholesterol (mg)	Total carb	Sugar (g)	Protein (g)	Calories
60	3	2	21	120
5	0	0	7	30
5	9	2	15	130
0	4	1	1	40

continued

Product flavor, serving size†	Approval	Nutrition or supplement		
		Total fat (g)	Sat. fat (g)	Sodium (mg)
Diet/Meal Replacement				
GNC Total Lean MRP™ Low-Glycemic Meal Replacement Formula, Chocolate, 48 g (1 packet)* Dist: General Nutrition Corporation	approved	2	0.5	250
Naturade® Total Soy® Meal Replacement, Bavarian Chocolate, serving size: 39 g (2 scoops) Dist: Naturade Inc.	approved	1	0	170
Nature's Plus® The Energy Supplements® Spiru-Tein® High Protein Energy Meal, Non-GMO Natural Soy®, Vanilla Soy Protein Powder with Spirulina, serving size: 34 g (1 scoop) Mf: Natural Organics Laboratories, Inc.	approved	0	0	140
Nestle® Carnation® Instant Breakfast® Nutritional Energy Drink for the Carb Conscious, Creamy Milk Chocolate Flavor, serving size: 315 mL (1 carton) Dist: Nestle USA, Inc.	approved	5	1.5	250

Cholesterol (mg)	Total carb	Sugar (g)	Protein (g)	Calories
5	30	5	9	180
0	20	16	14	140
0	11	8	14	99
10	15	12	12	150

continued

Product flavor, serving size†	Approval	Nutrition or supplement		
		Total fat (g)	Sat. fat (g)	Sodium (mg)
Slim-Fast® Optima™ 50% Less Sugar, Meal, Creamy Milk Chocolate Shake, serving size: 325 mL (1 can) Dist: Slim-Fast Foods Company	approved	5	1	220
Spirulina Soy Protein Drink, High Protein Soy Powder, Supro® Brand A Superior Protein, Rich & Creamy Vanilla Flavor, serving size: 33.6 g (1 scoop)* Mf: Vitamin World, Inc.	approved	0.5	0	200
Trim Advantage® Low Fat Drink Mix, Chocolate Flavor, serving size: 53 g (1 packet)* Dist: Access Business Group Intl. LLC	approved	2	0.5	340
Trim Advantage® Chocolate Caramel Flavored Ready To Go™ Meal Replacement Shake, serving size: 330 mL (1 carton)* Dist: Access Business Group Intl. LLC	approved	3	1	270

† Serving size listed in grams (g) for powders and milliliters (mL) for drinks. One fluid ounce is equal to approximately 30 mL.

‡ See also "More Brand Information," page 675.

*Tested through CL's Voluntary Certification Program before, at the time of, or after the initial review.

Cholesterol (mg)	Total carb	Sugar (g)	Protein (g)	Calories
5	24	17	10	180
0	16	14	14	120
5	30	21	15	170
<5	16	10	15	140

Part 7

Product Review: Articles

Breast Enhancement Supplements

Surgical breast enhancement is an enormous business in the United States; almost a quarter million such operations were performed in the year 2000 alone.[1] However, many women interested in breast augmentation are reluctant to undergo surgery, and would prefer to obtain the cosmetic results they desire in another way.

When there's a consumer need, entrepreneurs will step in to satisfy it. As a result, a bewildering variety of dietary supplements are advertised as effective breast size enhancers, complete with testimonials and scientific-sounding explanations for how they work.

ConsumerLab.com has received many inquiries about these supplements. As part of ConsumerLab.com's mission to identify better quality health and nutrition products, it first undertook a review of the scientific literature and information about the products on the market. This review concluded that there was no evidence to support the effective use of dietary supplements for breast enhancement. Consequently, CL saw no basis to proceed with laboratory testing of products as none could be recommended for breast enhancement.

Evidence For and Against Breast Enhancement Supplements

Two natural hormones, estrogen and progesterone, can increase breast size, but neither is a safe and effective medication for breast enlargement. Estrogen stimulates growth and development of breast tissue. If a woman takes extra estrogen, the glands and ducts in her breasts will be stimulated to grow, but only at an unacceptable cost: significantly increased risk of breast cancer. The hormone progesterone enlarges the breasts as well. However, it does so by stimulating milk-producing cells, hardly a viable option for nonpregnant women. Although estrogen and progesterone are found in prescription medications for gynecologic purposes, they are not approved for use in breast enhancement and not permitted to be sold as dietary supplements.

Numerous dietary supplements are marketed for breast enhancement, typically containing an assortment of herbal ingredients. Many Web sites describe studies in which all participants took a particular breast-enhancing product. Invariably, most of them reported benefit. However, such studies are virtually meaningless.

Human nature being what it is, people observe what they want to observe. In order to meaningfully evaluate the effectiveness of a proposed treatment for any condition, studies must be designed in such a way as to eliminate the power of suggestion.

Conducting what is called a double-blind, placebo-controlled trial does this. In such studies, half of the participants receive the treatment under study, and the other half receives a fake treatment (the placebo). Furthermore, both participants and researchers are kept in the dark about which group is which until the study has been completed. (Both groups are "blinded.") Double-blind studies eliminate the effect of the power of suggestion in all its many forms; only studies of this type can separate true effects from wishful thinking (or deliberate deception).

Unfortunately, there are no published double-blind studies on natural breast enhancement products. Some companies claim to possess evidence from double-blind studies that support their products, but, for some reason, do not wish to reveal their data. Thus, there is in fact no real evidence available that these products work.

Common Ingredients

Although there is little consistency in the detailed list of herbs and supplements contained in popular breast enhancement products, their ingredients tend to fall into four main categories:

- Phytoestrogens (such as soy, red clover, flaxseed, alfalfa, fennel, hops, licorice, turmeric, and verbena)

- Traditional aphrodisiacs (such as damiana and oat straw)

- Generic women's herbs (such as motherwort, blessed thistle, red raspberry, black cohosh, and chasteberry.)

- Miscellaneous herbs (such as saw palmetto, wild Mexican yam)

Aphrodisiacs and generic "women's herbs" are not really worth considering. Whether any herb acts as an aphrodisiac is a controversial matter, but it is beside the point. There's no particular reason an aphrodisiac should enlarge the breast.

Similarly, even though blessed thistle is traditionally regarded as helpful for menstrual pain, this does not imply that that it will help enlarge the breast.

The use of phytoestrogens for breast size enhancement, however, has at least a plausible basis. For this reason, we will examine it in detail. We will also look at two herbs in the miscellaneous category that are commonly included in breast enhancement products.

Phytoestrogens

Soybeans and numerous other plants contain substances called *phytoestrogens*. This term refers to naturally occurring chemicals that mimic the effects of estrogen. (See "Menopausal Symptom-Relief Supplements: Soy and Red Clover Isoflavones, Black Cohosh, and Progesterone Cream," page 116, volume 1.)

Phytoestrogens work by binding to certain docking sites on the cell membrane that are ordinarily used by estrogen. Technically, these docking sites are called *estrogen receptors*. When estrogen attaches to a receptor, it triggers a number of effects in the cell. Phytoestrogens can produce many of the same effects.

However, phytoestrogens don't bind to these receptors as perfectly as true estrogen does. Therefore, they produce a weaker effect on the cell. Furthermore, by physically attaching to these sites, phytoestrogens interfere with the ability of real estrogen to make contact with those sites. The net result is that phytoestrogens reduce estrogen's effects on the body. (NOTE: After menopause, the effect is somewhat different. Since the body is producing little estrogen, phytoestrogens may have a net positive effect on estrogen activity. But breast enhancement products are most often used by women who have not gone through menopause.)

This reduction of estrogenic action may be quite beneficial to a woman's health. By decreasing the effects of the body's own estrogen, phytoestrogens might reduce the chance of developing breast cancer, as well as other cancers that are stimulated by the presence of estrogen. This possibility has been advanced as an explanation for the low breast cancer rates in Asian countries, where soy is widely consumed.

Numerous natural products contain phytoestrogens. The most famous source is soy, but flaxseed, alfalfa, fennel, hops, licorice, red clover, turmeric, and verbena also contain reasonably high levels of estrogenic substances.[2]

Current evidence suggests that certain herbs once described as phytoestrogens may actually lack phytoestrogenic properties. These include dong quai,[2,3] ginseng,[4,5] and black cohosh[2,6-9]; however, black cohosh may have effects on menopausal symptoms through other mechanisms. The chastetree berry is also sometimes described as a source of phytoestrogen, but that is simply incorrect.

Phytoestrogens and Breast Size

Estrogen can increase breast size, although it is dangerous to use it for this purpose. Manufacturers of breast enhancement products claim that phytoestrogens also can enhance breast size, and safely. However, this hypothesis doesn't make any sense when you look at it closely.

As we just explained, phytoestrogens are much weaker than true estrogen, and at the same time they block the effects of true estrogen. Therefore, they should actually reduce estrogenic stimulation of the breast, not increase it.

Furthermore, breast enhancement products may not even contain much in the way of effective phytoestrogens. Two studies have evaluated the estrogenic powers of popular breast enhancement products, and found practically no phytoestrogenic action at all.[10,11]

In any case, if a breast enhancement product contained a phytoestrogen strong enough to stimulate breast growth, it would be too dangerous to use. As described earlier in this article, estrogen itself increases breast size, but only at the cost of increased cancer risk. Any phytoestrogen capable of stimulating breast growth would have the same dangerous side effect.

Other Herbs

The herb saw palmetto (often referred to as Sabal) is included in many breast enhancement formulas, apparently because of its traditional use for increasing milk production in nursing mothers.

Saw palmetto berries and berry extracts are best known as a treatment for prostate enlargement in men. It is not known precisely how saw palmetto works for this purpose, but it probably affects male sex hormones. Saw palmetto is not thought to have any estrogenic effects, and there is no scientific evidence that it affects breast size. (See "Prostate Health Supplements: Saw Palmetto and Beta-Sitosterol," page 162, volume 1.)

The herb wild Mexican yam is another popular ingredient in breast enhancement products, based on the widespread misconception that it contains progesterone. This common false belief probably stems from the role Mexican yam played in the history of hormone production. Mexican yam was used in the first commercially viable process for producing synthetic progesterone. It contains a substance called diosgenin, which organic chemists find handy as a starting point for synthesizing sex hormones. However, the body itself is unable to use diosgenin for that purpose. To all intents and purposes, Mexican yam is hormonally inactive.

Conclusion

There is neither good theoretical reason nor hard evidence to suggest that any natural breast enhancement product really works. Furthermore, if any such product actually did work, it would be too dangerous to use.

References

1. http://www.plasticsurgery.org/mediactr/qikfact1.pdf accessed 4/8/02

2. Zava DT, Dollbaum CM, Blen M. Estrogen and progestin bioactivity of foods, herbs, and spices. *Proc Soc Exp Biol Med.* 1998; 217: 369–378.

3. Hirata JD, Swiersz LM, Zell B, et al. Does dong quai have estrogenic effects in postmenopausal women? A double-blind, placebo controlled trial. *Fertil Steril.* 1997; 68: 981–986.

4. Forgo I, et al. The effect of a standardized ginseng extract on general well-being, reaction time, lung function and gonadal hormones. *Med Welt* 1981; 32: 751–756.

5. Wiklund IK, et al. Effects of a standardized ginseng extract on quality of life and physiological parameters in symptomatic postmenopausal women: a double-blind, placebo-controlled trial. Swedish Alternative Medicine Group. *Int J Clin Pharmacol Res* 1999;19: 89–99.

6. Einer-Jensen N, Zhao J, Andersen KP, et al. Cimicifuga and Melbosia lack oestrogenic effects in mice and rats. *Maturitas.* 1996; 25:149-153.

7. Jarry H, Harnischfeger G. Endocrine effects of constituents of *Cimicifuga racemosa*. 1. The effect on serum levels of pituitary hormones in ovariectomized rats. *Planta Med* 1985;1: 46–49.

8. Liske E. Therapeutic efficacy and safety of *Cimicifuga racemosa* for gynecologic disorders. *Adv Ther.* 1998;15: 45–53.

9. Nesselhut T Liske E. Pharmacological measures in postmenopausal women with an isopropanolic aqueous extract of Cimicifugae racemosae rhizoma. *Menopause* 1999; 1072–3714 6 Abst. #99.012.

10. Setchell KD, Brown NM, Desai P, et al. Bioavailability of pure isoflavones in healthy humans and analysis of commercial soy isoflavone supplements *J. Nutr.* 2001; 131: 362S–1375S.

11. Coldham NG, Sauer MJ. Identification, quantitation and biological activity of phytoestrogens in a dietary supplement for breast enhancement. *Food Chem.Toxicol.* 2001; 39: 1211–24.

Hoodia *(Hoodia gordonii)*

Hoodia *(Hoodia gordonii)* is a cactuslike succulent plant that grows in the high deserts of the Kalahari on the border of South Africa and Namibia. Hoodia is very rare and is protected by national conservation laws in South Africa and Namibia. Its stems and roots are used in supplements.

Stories claim that people indigenous to the Kalahari desert have used hoodia to stave off hunger during long-distance travel over the desert. In the 1960s, the Council for Scientific and Industrial Research (CSIR), a scientific research body in South Africa, included *Hoodia gordonii* among several hundred plant species in a project on edible wild plants. It found that rats fed hoodia lost weight but remained healthy.

One double-blind, placebo-controlled study of 18 obese people showed that those who took hoodia for 15 days ate 1,000 fewer calories daily, and burned more fat than those in the placebo group, without adverse effects. However, the study was fairly small and suspiciously has never been published in a peer-reviewed journal. Most of the other evidence for hoodia seems to be anecdotal, centering on personal experiences with the herb.

The ability of hoodia to suppress appetite or cause weight loss has been associated with a compound within the plant called P57, a steroidal alkaloid. One study found that injecting P57 into the brains of rats caused the animals to eat 40% to 60% less food. Researchers do not know whether the effect was due to the ingredient or other factors. However, P57 may work by increasing adenosine triphosphate (ATP) in nerve cells in the hypothalamus, the brain's control center for regulating thirst, temperature, and appetite. When levels of ATP are increased in hypothalamic nerve cells, those nerve cells fire, simulating the feeling that you have just eaten.

Interestingly, the drug company Pfizer began developing P57 as a prescription weight-control agent. However, in 2003 Pfizer discontinued clinical development of P57. The reason for this decision was not disclosed. More recently, the consumer products company Unilever (which makes Slim-Fast) announced that it had acquired the rights to develop and market hoodia as an ingredient in its weight-loss products.

Quality Concerns

There is some speculation that more hoodia is being sold today than could possibly be made from all the *Hoodia gordonii* plants in existence. Some of these products may be derived from other species of *Hoodia* or similar succulent plants from around the world. In such cases, consumers are likely not getting what they expect from the product.

In addition, no scientific standard presently exists for assessing the quality of hoodia as an ingredient, although attempts are being made to characterize its components. The quality of hoodia supplements, therefore, remains largely uncertain. As soon as a better characterization is available, ConsumerLab.com will likely purchase, test, and report on the quality of marketed products.

Dosages

Without published clinical trials to establish an optimal safe and effective dose, no one knows for certain how much hoodia should be taken. General dosing for hoodia is thought to be 3,000 to 4,000 mg a day of powder made from the roots and stems of *Hoodia gordonii* to trigger any sort of effect. Dosage for products made from concentrated extracts would be lower, depending on the concentration.

Interestingly, one popular weight-loss supplement, Trimspa, claims to contain hoodia (along with other ingredients) and suggests a daily dose that would yield only 500 mg of hoodia a day. Other manufacturers have different recommendations.

As with any weight-loss program, results will obviously be enhanced with a regimen that includes exercise and a reduced-calorie diet.

Concerns and Cautions

Although thought by some to be safe, safety studies have not been published for hoodia or P57. Further scientific studies are required to establish its safety.

Many supplements containing hoodia also have other weight-loss ingredients with potential side effects. Examples are bitter orange and caffeine, which can elevate heart rate and blood pressure, and can cause nervousness and sleeplessness.

Conclusion

Although tantalizing, the evidence for hoodia as a weight-loss ingredient remains anecdotal and preliminary, as does evidence of its safety. Whether the products on the market provide the authentic ingredient, whether the products recommend an appropriate dose, and whether using a hoodia supplement will help with weight loss are all also uncertain.

Noni Juice

Noni (*Morinda citrifolia*) is a small tree whose leaves, roots, bark, and fruit were traditionally used for topical ailments by a wide range of cultures across the Indian and Pacific Oceans. The word *noni* is from Polynesia, where much of the fruit is currently produced. During colonial times, the plant was taken to Africa, South America, and the Caribbean, where many local uses developed. Products specifically made from the juice of the noni fruit have been introduced into North America, Japan, and Europe in recent years.

Aside from its water content, noni fruit contains a large amount of carbohydrates, some protein, and a very small amount of fat. It also contains vitamin C, potassium, and smaller amounts of other vitamins and minerals. A variety of plant chemicals with possible biological activity have been reported in noni juice.

Traditionally, noni leaves, and not the fruit, have been used medicinally. The leaves have been employed as bandages for wounds or chopped and placed inside wounds. Roots and inner stem bark have been used for inflammatory and infectious conditions.

The immature fruit has been used occasionally for internal remedies, and the ripe fruit has been used as a poultice for wounds, skin infections, and to promote lactation. The ripe fruit has not generally been used orally as a medicine. Because of its strong odor, which has been described as vomitlike, the ripe fruit has not been regularly used as food other than during times of famine.

Much of the current usage of noni has little to do with traditional usage and focuses on the ripe fruit taken orally, as opposed to topically. Many current uses stem from an article in the *Pacific Tropical Botanical Garden Bulletin* in 1985 by Richard Heinicke. In the article, Heinicke claims that noni fruit contains a compound, proxeronine, that is converted into a compound called xeronine. He contends that xeronine is useful in treating high blood pressure, menstrual cramps, arthritis, gastric ulcers, sprains, injuries, mental depression, senility, poor digestion, drug addiction, and pain. The article also includes these claims (thought to be unsubstantiated or inaccurate):

- Noni must be taken on an empty stomach because a proenzyme that converts proxeronine to xeronine is susceptible to stomach acid.

- Cells contain proteins that have receptor sites for xeronine that also facilitate the activity of many active plant compounds.

- Noni is less effective and may have unexpected side effects if taken with caffeine, tobacco, or alcohol.

- Green fruit has more valuable components than ripe fruit.

Other modern claims say that noni juice is an immune system stimulant and is useful in AIDS, Epstein-Barr virus, cancer, lupus, and kidney problems. Noni has also been promoted for treating tuberculosis, diabetes, heart trouble, colds, influenza, counteracting side effects of kava, as a blood purifier, and as an insecticide for lice.

Evidence

Unfortunately, many of the claims made in Heinicke's 1985 article are thought to be inaccurate or unsubstantiated. In fact, the very existence of the compounds xeronine and proxeronine is questionable. Currently little scientific evidence exists to either support or refute the claims of noni's effectiveness.

Because of noni's popularity, however, scientists have begun studying noni in the laboratory. The results have been intriguing. The juice is thought to contain polysaccharides, which may have an immunostimulatory effect, and scopoletin (also found in tomatoes and chilies), which may dilate blood vessels and have other effects. Several in vitro studies have shown noni juice stimulates tumor necrosis factor and several interleukins, suppresses cell transformation and proliferation of breast and colon carcinomas, and induces apoptosis (programmed cell death). Researchers think that some of the compounds responsible for these effects are anthocyanins, which may emerge as useful compounds for testing the authenticity of noni products. Noni's leaves and roots contain other compounds with potential antibacterial and anticancer activity, but these plant parts are typically not sold as supplements.

Because of noni's potential anticancer activity and use by people with cancer, the National Institute of Health is funding a clinical study of dried noni fruit extract in cancer patients at the Cancer Research Center of Hawaii. The first phase will define noni's maximum tolerated dose and potential toxicities. It will also collect preliminary information on the efficacy of noni in respect to antitumor and symptom control. The study also seeks to identify chemical constituents of noni so that its bioavailability and pharmacokinetics can be measured and assessed.

Forms

Ripe or sub-ripe, undecomposed fruits are used to make preserved juice drinks, freeze-dried fruit juice, concentrated extracts, powders, tinctures, and fruit leather. There is controversy over which form is better. Fresh juice is sweeter and easier to drink because it contains more sugar. Aged juice, made by bacterial fermentation, is said to have a strong but mellow flavor. Water-added juice is made allowing the fruit to sit in water and is technically a fruit drink and not a juice. The NIH-sponsored clinical study is using pills, each containing 500 mg of freeze-dried noni extract.

Dosage

Manufacturers' recommendations range widely, as do the concentrations of noni in the products. Clinical trials have yet to establish the dose of noni fruit that is safe and effective in the treatment or prevention of any disease. However, it is thought that people can consume two to three fruits a day without problems.

Cautions

Noni is generally thought to be safe as a food. However, because noni is a plant in the coffee family, people with allergies or sensitivities to coffee may want to avoid using noni. Other related plant products that could involve cross-sensitivity include ipecac, quinine/quinidine, tonic water, gardenia oil, madder, and many natural red, orange or yellow dyes such as alizarin.

If you are counting calories or watching carbohydrate intake, be aware that noni juice, like other juices, may contribute both calories and carbohydrates to your diet.

The FDA has sent warning letters to several companies regarding unsubstantiated marketing claims, many of which repeat those made in Richard Heinicke's 1985 article. Products included in these warning letters in 2004 include Noni Juice Liquid Herbal Supplement, Noni Cleansing Formula AM/PM, and Pure Hawaiian Noni Juice.

Quality Concerns

Unlike most herbals sold as supplements, quality standards have yet to be defined for noni products. Currently, there is no way to judge whether one product is more effective or safe than another.

Reports suggest that some companies have sold the leftover by-products of juicing, for example, the discarded seed-pulp-fiber material, drying and grinding it and deceptively selling it as "100% noni fruit powder." Such a product would not contain the compounds expected in true noni juice. (However, there is no evidence that the fruit is better than the seeds, nor that the seeds are bad in any way.)

Noni has distinctive varieties and possibly even more than one species being used as the source of fruit. Almost all of the published literature is based upon fruit from trees in Hawaii. However, most of the fruit being sold is from trees growing in French Polynesia, Samoa, Fiji, and other South Pacific islands; the chemical constituents of these fruits may be different from the Hawaiian versions.

Noni fruit is often wild harvested (wild-crafted) and therefore may not have consistent quality nor origin.

Noni is also commercially grown and harvested. As with other commercially grown crops, pesticides may be used in its production. Noni fruit is often grown in countries where different laws regulate pesticide and herbicide usage, including chemicals that are no longer acceptable in the United States, Canada, or Europe. Some growers, however, do have organic certifications.

Some, but not all, noni juice is pasteurized. Pasteurization is a heat treatment intended to kill potential pathogens in food products and may prolong shelf life. Some researchers, however, argue that pasteurization might also inactivate compounds with potential beneficial effect, but such loss has not been proven.

Conclusion

Current usage of noni juice does not reflect its traditional usage and is driven predominantly by widely promoted claims that have yet to be substantiated or denied by clinical research. Laboratory research, however, suggests possible biological effects of noni juice. A clinical trial is under way to assess noni's effectiveness in cancer treatment and to better understand noni's chemical makeup.

Until more is known, it seems safe to use noni (other than potential allergic reaction), but its benefits remain unproven. The composition of noni products on the market may vary significantly because of a lack of standards and an optimal dosage has not been established.

References

Proceedings of the 2002 Hawai'i Noni Conference, S.C. Nelson (ed.), University of Hawaii at Manoa, College of Tropical Agriculture and Human Resources, 2003. Go to http://www.ctahr.hawaii.edu/noni/2002conference.asp.

McClatchey, W. From Polynesian healers to health food stores: Changing perspectives of *Morinda citrifolia* (Rubiaceae), *Integrative Cancer Therapies,* 1(2); 2002 PP. 110–220. Go to http://www.ctahr.hawaii.edu/noni/Downloads/MorindaCitrifolia.pdf.

For more information regarding the NIH clinical trial of noni, go to http://www.clinicaltrials.gov/show/NCT00033878.

Part 8

Product Screening

Products Screened for Substances Banned in Athletics

The Screening Program

ConsumerLab.com offers the Athletic Banned Substances Screening Program to test dietary supplements, performance enhancement products, and other nutrition products for substances that could cause athletes to be disqualified from Olympic and other competition. CL's program is the first comprehensive one to focus on supplements, as opposed to the downstream testing of body fluids from athletes. The ConsumerLab.com screening program includes testing supplements for banned substances, including stimulants, narcotics, anabolic agents, diuretics, masking agents, and beta-blockers based on the Olympic Movement Anti-Doping Code or the codes of other sports associations. This Screening Program is offered as an adjunct to ConsumerLab.com's Product Review testing.

Products That Passed Screening

Products that were screened for substances prohibited by the Olympic Movement Anti-Doping Code are listed alphabetically in Products That Passed Athletic Banned-Substance Screening. The ingredient categories for which the products were additionally tested are shown as well.

Products That Passed Athletic Banned-Substance Screening

Product (categories for which product was tested, identity and quality of prime ingredient)	Manufacturer (Mf) or distributor (Dist)	Date Tested
Amino Vital® FAST Charge Advance Amino Acid Sports Supplement*	Ajinomoto Co., Inc.	June 2004
Amino Vital® Lemon-Lime Flavor Advanced Amino Acid Sports Liquid Dietary Supplement*	Ajinomoto Co., Inc.	June 2004
Amino Vital® Mix and Shake*	Ajinomoto Co., Inc.	June 2004
Amino Vital® Orange Flavor Advanced Amino Acid Sports Liquid Dietary Supplement*	Ajinomoto Co., Inc.	June 2004
NITRO FX™, Noni whole plant extract Nitric oxide formula***	Enliven International, Inc.	May 2006
Pharmanex® LifePak® Dietary Supplement, New! Anti-Aging Formula (Alpha-Lipoic Acid, B Vitamins, Multivitamin, Vitamin C, Vitamin E)*	Pharmanex, LLC	December 2004
Tahitian Noni® Liquid Dietary Supplement**	Tahitian Noni International, Inc.	September 2005
XanGo™, Mangosteen supplement***	XanGo LLC	August 2006

Products Screened for Substances Banned in Athletics

*Testing based on World Anti-Doping Code Prohibited list available in 2004.
**Testing based on World Anti-Doping Code Prohibited list available in 2005.
***Testing based on World Anti-Doping Code Prohibited list available in 2006.

Appendices

ConsumerLab.com's Testing Methods and Standards

For each of the reviews, ConsumerLab.com evaluated the products using the best testing methods and standards available at the time. Consequently, many of the tests surpassed the requirements of the U.S. Food and Drug Administration (FDA). All products were tested to determine whether they contained the main ingredient specified on the label. On supplements known to have specific problems, additional tests were performed. Details of testing for each product review are given below.

Products passing ConsumerLab.com's evaluations had to meet specific criteria in either a first or second round of testing. Passing scores in each analysis included margins of technical error. In addition, ConsumerLab.com reserved the right to disqualify a product at any time if the product seemed to be unsafe or to provide misleading or inaccurate label information. Testing evolved over a three-year period, so methods and standards vary, depending on the time of the test.

The selection of products in all reviews represented those commonly sold or available nationally in the U.S. (and, in many cases, in Canada). ConsumerLab.com purchased products on the open market through retail stores, on-line retailers, catalogues, or multilevel marketing companies. Products were not accepted directly from manufacturers. For each product, the sample was composed of one or more purchased samples from a lot having an expiration date (if labeled) later than the date of testing.

Health Conditions

Bone-Health Supplements

Testing Methods: Calcium-containing products were tested for their amount of calcium as well as contamination with lead. Products with vitamin D were also tested for the form and amount of vitamin D. All tablets were tested for their ability to disintegrate (excluding chewable, time-release or extended-release forms).

Analyses for calcium and lead were performed using ICP-MS (Inductively Coupled Plasma-Mass Spectroscopy) method in an independent laboratory. Analysis for vitamin D utilized the USP extraction and HPLC methodology for finished products. Products not having passing levels of calcium, vitamin D, and lead were then retested on the failing parameter in a second independent laboratory using similar methods.

Disintegration of nonchewable, noncapsule, nonenteric-coated, and non-time-release formulations were analyzed utilizing USP (United States Pharmacopeia) <2040> recommendations entitled "Disintegration and Dissolution of Nutritional Supplements."

The identities of the products were not disclosed to the laboratories performing the testing.

Passing Score: To pass testing, a product had to meet the following criteria:

Calcium: Contain a minimum of 100% of its labeled amount of elemental calcium and not exceed 150% of this amount.

Not exceed California Prop 65 levels for lead contamination in a recommended daily serving and, in no event, exceed 2 mcg of lead in a recommended daily serving. (The State of California has established its own strict standards for lead, including 0.5 micrograms of lead per day for foods and most supplements. Calcium products providing 1,000 mg or more of elemental calcium per day have a limit of 1.5 micrograms (mcg) of lead. Products sold in California that exceed these levels are required to bear warning labels.)

Vitamin D: Contain a minimum of 100% of its labeled amount of total vitamin D and specific claims for vitamin D-2 or D-3 and not exceed 150% of these amounts.

All Products: Meet recommended USP parameters for disintegration for vitamin supplements (excluding capsule, enteric-coated, chewable, and time-release products).

Meet FDA labeling requirements.

A "Pass" was based on meeting the above criteria in either the first or second rounds of testing.

Cancer-Prevention Supplements

Testing Methods: The cancer prevention products were tested for amount(s) of selected key ingredients: green tea (*Camellia sinensis* L.), caffeine, lycopene, and selenium. Analyses included identification of potential contamination with lead in green tea products. All applicable products were also tested for their ability to disintegrate in solution (excluding capsules, chewable, and time-release products).

For each ingredient, these testing methods were employed.

Green tea: products were evaluated for specific forms: Total catechin concentration by HPLC and total green tea phenolics as gallic acid by Ultraviolet-Visible (UV-Vis) spectroscopy (Folin-Ciocalteu method). Green tea products were quantitatively analyzed for xanthine alkaloids (caffeine, theophylline, and theobromine) by HPLC. Lead contamination was assessed by ICP-MS analyses.

Selenium: Selenium products were analyzed using an Inductively Coupled Plasma-Mass Spectroscopy (ICP-MS) for total selenium and seleniomethionine forms as claimed or yeast content was measured by a special method.

Lycopene: Lycopene products were evaluated for cis-lycopene and total lycone content by HPLC.

All products: Disintegration of noncapsule, nonchewable, and non-time-release formulations was analyzed utilizing USP (United States Pharmacopeia) <2040> recommendations entitled "Disintegration and Dissolution of Nutritional Supplements."

Products not having passing levels of key ingredients or contaminants were then retested in a second independent laboratory using similar methods and instrumentation. The identities of the products were not disclosed to the laboratories performing the testing.

Passing Score: To achieve a "Pass" in the testing, a product had to meet the following criteria:

Green Tea Products: Contain a minimum of 100% and no more than 135% of label claim for total catechins or specific catechins (e.g., epigallocatechin gallate (EGCG)). Total catechins are the sum of epigallocatechin, epicatechin, epigallocatechin gallate, gallocatechin gallate, epicatechin gallate, and catechin gallate. Green tea extracts with no total catechin or specific catechin label claim should have no less than 10% total catechins (%wt/wt).

Contain no less than 100% and no more than 120% of label claim for xanthine alkaloids (as caffeine, theophylline, and theobromine).

Must not exceed California Prop 65 levels for lead contamination in a recommended daily serving and, in no event, exceed 2 mcg of lead in a recommended daily serving. (The State of California has established its own strict standards for lead, including 0.5 micrograms of lead per serving per day for foods and most supplements. Products sold in California that exceed these levels are required to bear warning labels.)

Selenium Products: Contain a minimum of 100% and no more than 135% of label claim of elemental selenium and seleniomethionine.

Lycopene Products: Contain a minimum of 100% and no more than 135% of label claim of total cis/trans lycopene or specific lycopene isomers.

All Products: Meet recommended USP parameters for disintegration for nutritional supplements (excluding capsule, chewable, and time-release products).

Meet FDA labeling requirements.

A product passed if it passed each criterion in any one of the analyses.

Cholesterol-Lowering Supplements

Testing Method: Guggulsterone, Policosanol, and Sterol products were subjected to the analyses listed below:

Guggulsterones: Quantitative Analysis of E and Z forms of guggulsterones performed by High Performance Liquid Chromatography HPLC with UV detection.

Analyses for lead and arsenic were performed using an ICP-MS (Inductively Coupled Plasma-Mass Spectroscopy) in an independent laboratory.

Policosanol: Quantitative Analysis of Policosanol by Gas Chromatography (GC) using a Flame Ionization Detector (FID) analytical method.

Sterols: Quantitative Analysis of Phytosterols by Gas Chromatography (GC) using a Flame Ionization Detector (FID) analytical method.

Disintegration of nonchewable, noncapsule, nonenteric-coated, and non-time-release formulations was analyzed utilizing USP (United States Pharmacopeia) <2040> recommendations entitled "Disintegration and Dissolution of Nutritional Supplements."

Any product that did not pass the testing was sent to another independent laboratory to repeat testing for at least one of the criteria on which it did not pass. The identities of the products were not disclosed to the laboratories performing the testing.

Passing Score: To pass testing, a product had to meet the following criteria:

Meet recommended USP parameters for disintegration for vitamin supplements (excluding capsule, enteric-coated, chewable, and time-release products).

Meet all FDA labeling requirements.

Guggulsterones: Must contain at least 100%, and not more than 150% of the claimed amount of total and specific guggulsterones.

The E and Z forms of guggulsterones must account for at least 2.5% and not more than 6.0% of the resin (extract) content if resin content is claimed.

Must not exceed CA Prop 65 levels for lead contamination in a recommended daily serving and, in no event, exceed 2 mcg of lead in a recommended daily serving and must not exceed 10 mcg of arsenic per suggested daily serving.

Policosanol: Must contain at least 100%, and not more than 150%, of its claimed amount of total policosanol.

The total policosanol must contain no less than 60% (%wt/wt) octacosanol. In addition, the sum of octacosanol, tetracosanol, hexacosanol, heptacosanol, triacosanol, and nonacosanol should represent no less than 85% (%wt/wt).

Sterols: Contain at least 100%, and not more than 150%, of its claimed amount of total plant sterol esters or free sterols.

If health claim is made, product must provide a minimum of 1.3 g total plant sterol esters divided over two or more servings per day (equivalent to a minimum of 0.813 g free sterols).

If product contains plant sterol esters, the sum of free beta-sitosterol, campesterol, and stigmasterol shall not be less than 62.5% of the total claimed amount.

A product passed testing if it met each applicable criterion in any one of the analyses.

Joint-Care Supplements

Testing Method: Products containing glucosamine or chondroitin were first analyzed by High Performance Liquid Chromatography (HPLC). Products that did not pass this initial test were reanalyzed in another independent laboratory using a HPLC method or capillary electrophoresis (CE) (for chondroitin).

Products containing MSM were tested for their claimed amount of MSM and for DMSO. Analysis for MSM and DMSO was performed using a Gas Chromatography (GC) method. Products not having passing levels of MSM or DMSO were then retested in a second independent laboratory using a comparable GC method.

Disintegration of nonchewable, noncapsule, nonenteric-coated, and non-time-release formulations were analyzed utilizing USP (United States Pharmacopeia) <2040> recommendations entitled "Disintegration and Dissolution of Nutritional Supplements."

Analyses for lead were performed using ICP-MS (Inductively Coupled Plasma-Mass Spectroscopy) method.

Analyses were conducted in independent laboratories to which the brand identities of the products were not disclosed. Any product not passing an initial analysis was retested in a second independent laboratory on at least one of the criteria it did not initially pass.

Passing Score: To pass testing, a product had to meet the following criteria:

Meet recommended USP parameters for disintegration for vitamin-mineral supplements (excluding capsule, enteric-coated, chewable, and time-release products).

Meet all FDA labeling requirements.

Glucosamine: Contain at least 100%, and not more than 150%, of claimed amount of the appropriate claimed form(s) of glucosamine.

Not exceed California Prop 65 levels for lead contamination in a recommended daily serving and, in no event, exceed 2 mcg of lead in a recommended daily serving. (The State of California has established its own strict standards for lead, including 0.5 micrograms of lead per day for foods and most supplements. Products sold in California that exceed these levels are required to bear warning labels.)

Chondroitin: Contain at least 100%, and not more than 150%, of claimed amount of total chondroitin.

MSM: Contain at least 100%, and not more than 125%, of claimed amount of MSM and less than 0.05% DMSO (%wt/wt).

Memory-Enhancement Supplements

Testing Methods: Products were tested for amount(s) of selected key ingredients: acetyl-L-carnitine, ginkgo biloba, huperzine A, and phosphatidylserine. Analyses included identification of potential contamination with lead in botanical products. The products were also tested for their ability to disintegrate in solution (excluding capsules, chewable and time-release products).

For each ingredient, the following testing method was employed:

Acetyl-L-carnitine: Quantitative analysis of acetyl-L-carnitine by High Performance Liquid Chromatography (HPLC) using Ultra Violet (UV) detection.

Ginkgo: Quantitative analysis of bilobalide and ginkgolides (Terpene Lactones) by HPLC using an Evaporative Light Scattering Detector (ELSD) or by a Gas Chromatographic (GC) method.

Quantitative analysis of flavonol glycosides utilizing a HPLC method with UV detection.

Analyses for lead were performed using Inductively Coupled Plasma-Mass Spectroscopy (ICP-MS) instrumentation.

Huperzine A: Quantitative analysis of (-) huperzine A performed by Capillary Electrophoresis (CE) with UV detection.

Analyses for lead were performed using an Inductively Coupled Plasma-Mass Spectroscopy (ICP-MS).

Phosphatidylserine: Quantitative analysis of phosphatidylserine performed by HPLC-UV.

Disintegration of nonchewable, noncapsule, nonenteric-coated and non-time-release formulations was analyzed utilizing USP (United States Pharmacopeia) <2040> recommendations entitled "Disintegration and Dissolution of Nutritional Supplements."

Analyses were conducted in an independent laboratory to which the brand identities of the products were not disclosed. Any products not passing the initial analyses was retested in a second independent laboratory on at least one of the criteria it did not initially pass.

Passing Score: To pass testing, a product had to meet the following criteria: Meet recommended USP parameters for disintegration for nutritional supplements (excluding capsule, chewable, and time-release products). Meet all FDA labeling requirements.

A product passed if it passed each criterion in any one of the analyses.

Acetyl-L-carnitine: Contain a minimum of 100% and not exceed 150% of label claim for acetyl-L-carnitine (free base) or acetyl-L-carnitine complexes (e.g. acetyl-L-carnitine hydrochloride).

Ginkgo: State a recommended daily dosage on its label that would provide a clinically appropriate amount of ginkgo biloba leaf extract.

Contain at least 100%, and not more than 150% of the expected amounts of total and individual flavonol glycosides and total terpene lactones based on the claimed amount of ginkgo biloba leaf extract and the ratios defined as follows.

Flavonol Glycosides:

Total flavonol glycosides 22-27% (wt/wt)** (Sum of quercetin, kaempferol, and isorhamnetin)

Quercetin	minimum 9.5% (wt/wt)
Kaempferol	minimum 10.5% (wt/wt)
Isorhamnetin	minimum 2.0% (wt/wt)

Terpene Lactones:
Total terpene lactones 5-7% (wt/wt)** (Sum of ginkgolides A,B,C and bilobalide)

Ginkgolides A, B, C	minimum 2.8%(wt/wt)**
Bilobalide	minimum 2.6% (wt/wt)**

**Reference: German Commission E Monograph, American Herbal Pharmacopoeia Monograph

Not exceed California Prop 65 levels for lead contamination in a recommended daily serving and, in no event, exceed 2 mcg of lead in a recommended daily serving. (The State of California has established its own strict standards for lead, including 0.5 micrograms of lead per serving per day for foods and most supplements. Products sold in California that exceed these levels are required to bear warning labels.)

Huperzine A: State a recommended daily dosage on its label that would provide a clinically appropriate amount of (-) - huperzine A.

Contain at least 100% and not more than 150%, of the expected amount of (-) - huperzine A. If product claims to be made from natural source huperzine A (e.g., *Huperzia serrata* (Thunb. ex Murray) Trevis, toothed club moss) the expected amount of (-) - huperzine A shall be equivalent to the claimed amount of huperzine A. If product does not claim to be from natural source, or claims to be made from synthetic huperzine A, 50% of the claimed amount of huperzine A shall be expected to be (-) - huperzine A.

Not exceed California Prop 65 levels for lead contamination in a recommended daily serving and, in no event, exceed 2 mcg of lead in a recommended daily serving. (The State of California has established its own strict standards for lead, including 0.5 micrograms of lead per serving per day for foods and most supplements. Products sold in California that exceed these levels are required to bear warning labels.)

Phosphatidylserine: Contain a minimum of 100% and not exceed 150% of label claim for phosphatidylserine.

Menopause Symptom-Relief Supplements

Testing Methods: Soy, red clover, and combination products were tested for their total isoflavone content (specifically glycosidic and aglycone forms of the isoflavones). All products were analyzed using a HPLC (High Performance Liquid Chromatography) assay in an independent laboratory. The extraction and HPLC method was designed to specifically test for the presence and amount of various glycosidic and aglycone forms of the isoflavones found in soy and red clover. Products not passing this initial assay were tested in a second independent laboratory utilizing a similar HPLC assay.

Progesterone cream products were tested for their progesterone content and for potential contamination with other steroids. Products were analyzed by GC/MS/MS for progesterone content and for undeclared steroidal ingredients. Products not passing this initial assay for progesterone were tested in a second independent laboratory using a method from USP 28, NF 23.

Products containing Black Cohosh were evaluated for triterpene glycoside content (using 23-*epi*-26-deoxyactein as a standard) by HPLC-ELSD according to the INA method (113.001) and a published, modified USP method.

Disintegration of nonchewable and nontime release formulations was analyzed utilizing USP (United States Pharmacopeia) <2040> recommendations entitled "Disintegration and Dissolution of Nutritional Supplements."

All testing was conducted in independent laboratories to which the identities of the products were not disclosed.

Passing Score: To achieve a "Pass" in the testing, a product had to meet applicable criteria:

Soy and Red Clover Isoflavones: Meet 100% of label claim for total isoflavone content and, if declared, for specific glycosidic or aglycone isoflavones. Total isoflavones is calculated as the sum of the glycosidic and aglycone forms.

Black Cohosh: Meet 100% of label claim for total triterpene glycosides, and not more than 150% of the claim

Contain a minimum of 1 mg of total triterpene glycosides per daily recommended dose. An "extract" product must also contain a minimum of 2.5% triterpene glycosides. (Reference: German Commission E Expanded Monographs recommends 40 mg of extract standardized to 2.5% triterpene glycosides per day.)

Progesterone Creams : Meet 100% of label claim for progesterone, and not more than 125% of the claim. Not contain unlisted steroidal compounds that, in total, exceed 1% of the total progesterone found in the product (% wt/wt).

All Products: Meet recommended USP parameters for disintegration for vitamin supplements (excluding chewable and time-release products).

Meet all FDA labeling requirements.

For a product to fail, confirmation of a failing result was required on at least one of the criteria through repeat testing in a second independent laboratory.

Muscular-Enhancement Supplements

Testing Method:

Creatine: Creatine products were tested for their amount of creatine monohydrate or phosphate and potential contamination with creatinine and dicyandiamide. All creatine products were subjected to High Performance Liquid Chromatography (HPLC) to analyze for creatine as well as for creatinine and dicyandiamide. The HPLC methods employed are widely used in the industry and were internally verified.

HMB: Quantitative analysis of HMB was performed by High Performance Liquid Chromatography (HPLC) with UV detection.

Glutamine: Quantitative analysis of L-glutamine was performed by High Performance Liquid Chromatography (HPLC) with UV detection.

Amino Acids: Quantitative analyses for amino acids were performed before and after hydrolysis by an Amino Acid Analyzer.

Disintegration of nonchewable, noncapsule, nonenteric-coated, and non-time-release formulations were analyzed utilizing USP (United States Pharmacopeia) <2040> recommendations entitled "Disintegration and Dissolution of Nutritional Supplements."

Any product that did not pass the testing was sent to another independent laboratory to repeat testing for at least one of the criteria on which it did not pass. The identities of the products were not disclosed to the laboratories performing the testing.

Passing Score: To pass testing, a product had to meet the following criteria:

All products had to meet recommended USP parameters for disintegration for vitamin supplements (excluding capsule, enteric-coated, chewable, and time-release products) and all FDA labeling requirements.

Creatine: Must contain not less than 99.9% of the claimed amount of creatine monohydrate or phosphate.

The combined weights of creatinine and dicyandiamide found in the product could not represent more than 0.1% of the measured weight of the creatine monohydrate or phosphate.

HMB: Must contain at least 100%, and not more than 150%, of the claimed amount of total HMB.

Glutamine: Must contain at least 100%, and not more than 150%, of the claimed amount of total L-glutamine.

Amino Acids: Must contain at least 100%, and not more than 150%, of the claimed amount of individual and total amino acids.

A "Pass" was based on passing each criterion in any one of the analyses or laboratories.

Nuclear Radiation Protection Supplements

Testing Methods: Products were tested for the ability to disintegrate and the amount of iodine. Analyses for iodine were first performed ICP-MS (Inductively Coupled Plasma-Mass Spectroscopy) in an independent laboratory. Products not having passing levels of iodine were then retested in a second independent laboratory using the similar methods and instrumentation. The identities of the products were not disclosed to the laboratories performing the testing.

Disintegration of nonchewable, noncapsule, nonenteric-coated, and non-time-release formulations was analyzed utilizing USP (United States Pharmacopeia) <2040> recommendations entitled "Disintegration and Dissolution of Nutritional Supplements."

Passing Score: To pass testing, a product had to do the following.

Have a minimum of 92.5% of its labeled amount of elemental iodine and a maximum of 107.5% of this amount. (USP 25 official monograph; potassium iodide tablets)

Meet recommended USP parameters for disintegration.

A product passed if it passed each criterion in any one of the analyses.

Prostate-Health Supplements

Testing Methods: Saw palmetto products were tested for their total fatty acid and sterol content, while beta-sitosterol products were tested for their sterol content. All products were first analyzed for their respective constituents using a Gas Chromatography (GC) assay in an independent laboratory. Products not passing this initial assay were tested in a second independent laboratory utilizing a similar GC assay.

The identities of the products were not disclosed to the laboratories performing the testing.

Passing Score: To pass testing, a product had to meet the following criteria:

Saw Palmetto: Recommend a daily dosage on its label that would provide at least 320 mg of saw palmetto berry extract containing at least 85% fatty acids and sterols, 800 mg of a dried extract containing approximately 25% fatty acids and sterols, or one to two grams of saw palmetto berry powder.** Contain a minimum of 100%, and not more than 150%, of the expected amounts of total or individual fatty acids and total or individual sterols from the berry extract based on the claimed amount of saw palmetto berry extract and the ratios defined in fatty acids.*

Fatty Acids

Total Fatty Acids: 85 to 95%*(%wt/wt.)**
(Sum of fatty acids below)

Individual Fatty Acids:***	Formula	Percentage
Caproic Acid	$C_6H_{12}O_2$	1.0-3.0
Caprylic Acid	$C_8H_{16}O_2$	1.0-3.0
Capric Acid	$C_{10}H_{20}O_2$	1.0-3.0
Lauric Acid	$C_{12}H_{24}O_2$	25.0-32.0
Myristic Acid	$C_{14}H_{28}O_2$	10.0-15.0
Palmitic Acid	$C_{16}H_{32}O_2$	7.0-11.0
Stearic Acid	$C_{18}H_{36}O_2$	1.0-2.0
Oleic Acid	$C_{18}H_{34}O_2$	26.0-35.0
cis-Linoleic Acid	$C_{18}H_{32}O_2$	3.0-5.0
Linolenic Acid	$C_{18}H_{30}O_2$	0.5-1.5

Total Sterols: 0.2% (%wt/wt)(sum of campesterol, stigmasterol, and beta-sitosterol)***
Individual Sterols***

Campesterol	$C_{28}H_{48}O$	0.01-0.1
Stigmasterol	$C_{29}H_{48}O$	0.01-0.1
Beta-sitosterol	$C_{29}H_{50}O$	0.1-0.4

*For products containing berry powder only and no extract, the total and individual constituents were calculated as 10% (w/w) of the extract values. For products containing 25% dried extract, the total and individual constituents were calculated as 2.9.4% (w/w) of the 85% extract values.
**Based on German Commission E monograph.
***Based on industry specification standards.

Beta-sitosterol: Must contain a minimum of 100%, and not more than 150%, of the claimed amounts of beta-sitosterol and individual claimed sterols.

All Products: Meet recommended USP parameters for disintegration for vitamin supplements (excluding capsule, enteric-coated, chewable, and time-release products). Had to meet FDA labeling requirements.

A "Pass" was based on meeting the above criteria in either the first or second rounds of testing.

Sexual-Enhancement Supplements

Testing Methods: L-arginine products were tested for their total L-arginine content, while yohimbe products were tested for their yohimbine or total yohimbe alkaloid content and epimedium products were tested for their icariin content. All products were first analyzed for their respective constituents using a High Performance Liquid Chromatography (HPLC) assay in an independent laboratory. Arginine and yohimbe products were assayed utilizing USP Monograph methods. Products not passing this initial assay were tested in a second independent laboratory utilizing a similar HPLC assay.

All products were tested for sildenafil citrate, tadalafil, and vardenaifil or their analogs by HPLC/MS/MS.

The identities of the products were not disclosed to the laboratories performing the testing.

Passing Score: To pass testing, a product had to meet the following criteria.

L-Arginine: Had to meet 100% of label claim for L-arginine (free base) or L-arginine complexes (e.g., arginine hydrochloride).

Yohimbe: Provide all of the following information in its labeling for yohimbe (as required by the FDA)—

The proper plant name (Yohimbe; *Pausinystalia johimbe* K. Schum. or *Corynanthe yohimbe* K. Schum.);

The part of the plant used (bark);

The form of yohimbe used (e.g., bark powder or bark extract);

The amount of yohimbe bark powder or bark extract per pill or amount in grams (g) or milligrams (mg) [1 gram = 1,000 milligrams].

Contain a minimum of 100% and not exceed 135% of label claim for yohimbine or total yohimbe alkaloid content, with a minimum of of 0.19% of yohimbine and 2.7% total yohimbe alkaloids for bark powder preparations.

Epimedium: Provide all of the following information in its labeling for yohimbe (as required by the FDA)—

The proper plant name (Barrenwort or Epimedium; *Epimedium grandiflorum* Morr. (barrenwort), *Epimedium brevicornum* Maxim. (epimedium), *Epimedium koreanum* Nakai (epimedium), *Epimedium sagittatum*);

The part of the plant used (dried aerial part of the plant (leaves and some stems/stalks));

The form of epimedium used (e.g., powder or extract);

The amount of epimedium powder or extract per pill or dose in grams (g) or milligrams (mg) [1 gram = 1,000 milligrams]

Contain a minimum of 100% of label claim for icariin or if a claim is not made, a minimum of 1% icariin for aerial plant powder (Pharmacopeia People's Republic of China, English edition, 1997).

All Products: Must not contain any amount of sildenafil citrate, tadalafil, and vardenaifil or their analogs. Had to meet FDA labeling requirements.

A "Pass" was based on meeting the above criteria in either the first or second rounds of testing.

Sight-Enhancement Supplements

Testing Method: Products were tested for their claimed amount of lutein and zeaxanthin. Analysis for lutein and zeaxanthin was performed using an HPLC method in an independent laboratory. Products not having passing levels of lutein and zeaxanthin were then retested in a second independent laboratory using a similar HPLC method.

Disintegration of nonchewable, noncapsule, nonenteric-coated and non-time-release formulations were analyzed utilizing USP (United States Pharmacopeia) <2040> recommendations entitled "Disintegration and Dissolution of Nutritional Supplements."

Analyses were conducted in independent laboratories to which the brand identities of the products were not disclosed. Any product not passing an initial analysis was retested in a second independent laboratory on at least one of the criteria on which it did not initially pass.

Passing Score: To pass testing, a product had to meet the following criteria:

Contain at least 100% of its labeled amount of lutein and zeaxanthin and no more than 150% of this amount.

Meet recommended USP parameters for disintegration for vitamin supplements (excluding capsule, enteric-coated, chewable, and time-release products).

Meet all FDA labeling requirements.

A product passed if it passed each applicable criterion in any one of the analyses.

Weight-Loss and Slimming Supplements

Testing Methods: The weight-loss products were tested for amount(s) of selected key ingredients: bitter orange (sour orange, *Citrus aurantium* L.), 7-keto DHEA, green tea (*Camellia sinensis* L.), hydroxycitric acid (HCA), caffeine, chromium, and pyruvate. Analyses included identification of potential contamination with hexavalent chromium in chromium products, lead in botanical products, and undeclared stimulants in stimulant-containing products. The products were also tested for their ability to disintegrate in solution (excluding capsules, chewable, and time-release products).

For each ingredient, the following testing method was employed:

7-keto-dehydroepiandrosterone (7-keto DHEA or 7-keto): 7-keto DHEA products were analyzed by HPLC.

Bitter orange: Bitter orange products were quantitatively analyzed for synephrine-type alkaloids (synephrine, hordenine, N-methyl tyramine, octopamine, tyramine) by High Performance Liquid

Chromatography (HPLC), Capillary Electrophoresis (CE), and screened by Gas Chromatography with Mass Spectral Detection (GC-MS).

Chromium: Chromium products were analyzed using an Inductively Coupled Plasma-Mass Spectroscopy (ICP-MS) for total chromium and Ion Chromatography (EPA method 3060A/7199) for hexavalent chromium (chromium VI).

Green tea: Green tea products were evaluated for catechin concentration by HPLC and total green tea phenolics as gallic acid by Ultraviolet-Visible (UV-Vis) spectroscopy (Folin-Ciocalteu method).

Hydroxycitric acid (HCA): Hydroxycitric acid products were analyzed by High Performance Liquid Chromatography (HPLC).

Pyruvate: Pyruvate products were analyzed for their pyruvate content by HPLC and Capillary Electrophoresis (CE). Dihydroxyacetone in pyruvate products were analyzed by HPLC.

Other tests: Any product claiming to contain bitter orange or a stimulant blend was screened for stimulants and related compounds by Gas Chromatography. Confirmation of any detected stimulant substances was made by GC-mass spectroscopy. Products were quantitatively analyzed for synephrine-type alkaloids and xanthine alkaloids (caffeine, theophylline, and theobromine) by HPLC.

Disintegration of noncapsule, nonchewable, and non-time-release formulations was analyzed utilizing USP (United States Pharmacopeia) <2040> recommendations entitled "Disintegration and Dissolution of Nutritional Supplements."

Lead was analyzed by ICP-MS.

Products not having passing levels of key ingredients or contaminants were then retested in a second independent laboratory using similar methods and instrumentation. The identities of the products were not disclosed to the laboratories performing the testing.

Passing Score: To achieve a "Pass" in the testing, a product had to meet the following criteria:

7-Keto: Contain no less than 100% and no more than 135% of label claim of 7-keto.

Bitter orange and stimulant blends: Contain a minimum 100% and no more than 135% of label claim for synephrine and contain other bitter orange alkaloids (hordenine, N-methyl tyramine, octopamine, tyramine) in appropriate levels 4:1. Dry extracts without label claim should have no less than 1% synephrine and no more than 6% (%wt/wt of peel extract) and contain other bitter orange alkaloids (hordenine, N-methyl tyramine, octopamine, tyramine) in appropriate levels 4:1.

Contain 100% and no more than 120% of label claim for xanthine alkaloids (as caffeine, theophylline, and theobromine).

Contain no detectable amounts of stimulants if the products did not claim to contain caffeine, stimulants, or related ingredients.

Chromium: Contain a minimum of 100% and no more than 120% of label claim for total chromium.

Contain less than 0.1% of hexavalent chromium (chromium VI) by %wt/wt of total chromium.

Green tea: Contain a minimum of 100% and no more than 135% of label claim for total catechins or specific catechins (e.g. epigallocatechin gallate (EGCG)). Total catechins are the sum of epigallocatechin, epicatechin, epigallocatechin gallate, gallocatechin gallate, epicatechin gallate, and catechin gallate. Green tea extracts with no total catechin or specific catechin label claim should have no less than 10% total catechins (%wt/wt).

Contain no less than 100% and no more than 120% of label claim for xanthine alkaloids (as caffeine, theophylline, and theobromine).

HCA: Contain a minimum of 100% and no more than 135% of label claim of HCA.

Pyruvate: Contain a minimum of 100% and no more than 135% of label claim of pyruvate and dihydroxyacetone.

All Products: Must not exceed California Prop 65 levels for lead contamination in a recommended daily serving and, in no event, exceed 2 mcg of lead in a recommended daily serving. (The State of California has established its own strict standards for lead, including 0.5 micrograms of lead per serving per day for foods and most supplements. Products sold in California that exceed these levels are required to bear warning labels.)

Meet recommended USP parameters for disintegration for nutritional supplements (excluding capsule, chewable, and time-release products).

Meet all FDA labeling requirements.

A product passed if it passed each criterion in any one of the analyses.

Herbal Products

Asian and American Ginseng

Testing Method: Ginseng products were tested for their amount of total ginsenosides and potential contamination with specific heavy metals and pesticides. Analysis for ginsenosides was made by High

Performance Liquid Chromatography (HPLC) using the Ginseng Evaluation Program (GEP) methods established by the American Botanical Council (ABC). This analysis specifically tests for the presence and amount of the seven major types of ginsenosides. Based on the scientific literature, the weight of these seven ginsenosides is assumed to represent approximately 90% of the total ginsenosides in a product and is therefore used to calculate the total ginsenoside weight in products.

Analyses for the heavy metals arsenic, cadmium, and lead were made using Inductively Coupled Plasma/Mass Spectroscopy (ICP/MS).

Analysis for the pesticides quintozene (pentachloronitrobenzene), lindane (hexachlorocyclohexane), hexachlorobenzene and related compounds (pentachloroaniline, pentachlorothioanisol, alpha-benzenehexachloride, beta-benzenehexachloride, delta-benzenehexachloride, and tetrachloroanaline) was performed using a modified method by High Resolution Gas Chromatography (HRGC) with an electron capture detector (ECD) and High Resolution Gas Chromatography (HRGC) with mass spectroscopy/mass spectroscopy (MS/MS) detection described in the U.S. FDA Pesticide Analytical Manual (PAM) and a modification of the PAM method (presented at the September 1999 AOAC, Houston, Texas, entitled "Trace Contaminants in Dietary Supplements: Pesticide Analysis in Ginseng").

Analysis for caffeine, theobromine, and theophylline was done by HPLC.

Disintegration of nonchewable, noncapsule, nonenteric-coated and non-time-release formulations was analyzed utilizing USP (United States Pharmacopeia) <2040> recommendations entitled "Disintegration and Dissolution of Nutritional Supplements."

Any product that did not pass the testing was sent to another independent laboratory to repeat testing for at least one of the criteria on which it did not pass. The identities of the products were not disclosed to the laboratories performing the testing.

Passing Score: To achieve a "Pass" in the testing, a product had to meet the following criteria:

Meet its label claims for ginsenoside content and, at a minimum, contain the following total ginsenosides, respective of the type of ginseng labeled: 1.5% for Asian root powder (German Commission E recommendation), 3.0% for Asian root extract (USP recommendations), 2.0% for American root powder, and 4.0% for American root extract (common industry standard).

Heavy Metal Contamination: Must not exceed California Prop 65 levels for lead contamination in a recommended daily serving and, in no event, exceed 2 mcg of lead in a recommended daily serving. (The State of California has established its own strict standards for lead, including 0.5 micrograms of lead per serving per day for foods and most supplements—although this is raised to 1.5 micrograms per daily serving for calcium supplements. Products sold in California that exceed these levels are required to bear warning labels.) Contain less than 0.3 parts per million (or micrograms per gram of dried root) of cadmium (World Health Organization proposed guidelines). Contain less than 10 micrograms of arsenic per daily serving (state of California).

Pesticide Contamination: Contain less than 0.1 part per million of hexachlorobenzene, 1 part per million of quintozene (total of pentachloronitrobenzene (PCNB), pentachloroaniline, and pentachlorothioanisol), and less than 0.6 part per million of lindane (United States Pharmacopeia/European Pharmacopeia).

Caffeine levels in the product must not exceed those expected from declared ingredients.

Meet recommended USP parameters for disintegration for vitamin supplements (excluding capsule, enteric-coated, chewable, and time-release products).

Meet all FDA labeling requirements.

Echinacea

Testing Methods: Echinacea products were tested for their phenolic content (specifically caftaric acid, chlorogenic acid, echinacoside and cichoric acid), potential contamination with microbes, lead, and cadmium, and their ability to disintegrate (break apart) properly.

All products were first analyzed in an independent laboratory for the phenolic constituents utilizing a HPLC (High Performance Liquid Chromatography) assay developed by the Institute for Nutraceutical Advancement's (INA) Method Validation Program (MVP) to specifically test for the presence and amount of caftaric acid, chlorogenic acid, echinacoside and cichoric acid. Products not passing this initial assay were tested in a second independent laboratory using the same HPLC method.

Analyses for microbial contaminants were made using methods from the FDA's Bacteriological Analytical Manual (BAM) and included testing for *Escherichia coli, Salmonella* spp. *Staphylococcus aureus,*

Pseudomonas aeruginosa and other enteric bacteria including *Klebsiella, Enterobacter, Proteus, Citrobacter, Aerobacter, Providencia,* and *Serratia.* Testing also included analyses for total aerobic bacteria, yeast, and mold. Any product that did not pass the microbial testing was sent to another independent laboratory to repeat testing for any of the microbial criteria for which it did not pass.

Analyses for the heavy metals cadmium and lead were made using Inductively Coupled Plasma/Mass Spectroscopy (ICP/MS) or Atomic Absorption/Graphite Furnace.

Disintegration of nonchewable, noncapsule, nonenteric coated and nontime-release formulations was analyzed utilizing USP (United States Pharmacopeia) <2040> recommendations entitled "Disintegration and Dissolution of Nutritional Supplements."

Any product that did not pass the testing was sent to another independent laboratory to repeat testing for at least one of the criteria on which it did not pass. The identities of the products were not disclosed to the laboratories performing the testing.

Passing Score: To achieve a "Pass" in the testing, a product had to meet the following criteria:

Provide all of the following information in its labeling (as required by the FDA):

–The species of echinacea (i.e., *E. purpurea, E. angustifolia,* or *E. pallida*);

–The part of the plant used, such as root or the aerial (aboveground) portions which include the stem, leaves, and flowers and is also generally referred to as the "herb";

–The form of echinacea used (e.g., whole herb or root, extract, or tincture);

–The amount of echinacea per pill or dose in grams (g) or milligrams (mg) [1 gram = 1,000 milligrams]

Meet its label claims for total phenolic content, with a minimum of 1.0% total phenols based on whole herb or root, or proportionally higher for extracts or tinctures depending on their level of concentration. Total phenols were calculated as the sum of caftaric acid, chlorogenic acid, echinacoside, and cichoric acid.

Products labeled as containing the roots of *E. angustifolia* and *E. pallida* were required to contain the specific marker compound echinacoside and low levels of cichoric acid; products labeled to contain roots or herb of *E. purpurea* were required to contain cichoric, caftaric, and chlorogenic acids but, if they were *E. purpurea*–only products, could not have more than trace levels of echinacoside.

Test negative for *Escherichia coli, Salmonella* spp., *Staphylococcus aureus,* and *Pseudomonas aeruginosa* (as required by the FDA). In addition, contain less than the following levels of microbes per gram (as specified by the World Health Organization, Quality Control Methods for Medicinal Plant Material, 1998):
   –100,000 aerobic bacteria
   –1,000 yeast and mold
   –1,000 other coliform bacteria
Not exceed California Prop 65 levels for lead contamination in a recommended daily serving and, in no event, exceed 2 mcg of lead in a recommended daily serving.

Contain less than 0.3 parts per million (or micrograms per gram) of cadmium for dried raw herb (World Health Organization, Quality Control Methods for Medicinal Plant Material, proposed guidelines, 1998) or less than 0.1 parts per million for extracts. The lower concentration standard for extracts reflects the ability to remove heavy metals such as cadmium during the extraction process.

Meet recommended USP parameters for disintegration for vitamin supplements (excluding capsule, enteric-coated, chewable, and time-release products).

A "Pass" was based on meeting the above criteria in either the first or second rounds of testing.

Garlic

Testing Method: Garlic products with label claims for their alliin content, allicin yield and other related compounds were tested for the various constituents, while garlic products making no label claims were tested for their alliin content, allicin yield or gamma-glutamyl-(S)-allyl-L-cysteine content. All products were first analyzed using USP Monograph methods utilizing a HPLC (High Performance Liquid Chromatography) assay in an independent laboratory.

Disintegration of nonchewable, noncapsule, nonenteric coated and nontime-release formulations were analyzed utilizing USP (United States Pharmacopeia) <2040> recommendations entitled "Disintegration and Dissolution of Nutritional Supplements."

Analyses for the heavy metals arsenic, cadmium, and lead were made using Inductively Coupled Plasma/Mass Spectroscopy (ICP/MS).

Any product that did not pass the testing was sent to another independent laboratory to repeat testing for at least one of the criteria on which it did not pass. The identities of the products were not disclosed to the laboratories performing the testing.

Passing Score: To achieve a "Pass" in the testing, a product had to meet the following criteria:

Meet 100% of label claims for alliin, allicin yield, alliinase activity, total gamma-glutamylcysteines and gamma-glutamyl-(S)-allyl-L-cysteine;

If no label claim was made for garlic constituents, product had to meet the minimum marker levels for the specific garlic type in the product:

- Fresh or dried garlic products, of Allium sativum Linne, had to contain not less than 0.5% alliin and not less than 0.2% gamma-glutamyl-(S)-allyl-L-cysteine calculated on the dry weight basis. (USP 25 Official Monograph)
- Aged garlic, prepared from the fresh or dried bulbs of Allium sativum Linne, had to contain not less than 0.05% gamma-glutamyl-(S)-allyl-L-cysteine calculated on the dry weight basis.
- Powdered garlic, from dried or freeze-dried bulbs of Allium sativum Linne, had to contain not less than 0.3% alliin and not less than 0.1% gamma-glutamyl-(S)-allyl-L-cysteine calculated on the dry weight basis. (USP 25 Official Monograph)
- Powdered garlic extract, from the fresh bulbs of Allium sativum Linne, hd to contain not less than 4.0% alliin calculated on a dry weight basis. (USP 25 Official Monograph)
- Fresh or dried, powdered or powdered garlic extract containing products had to meet label claim for allicin potential and produce no less than 3,000 mcg allicin/g garlic (dry wt.).

Suggested daily dose of nonaged garlic products had to yield at least 2,400 mcg of allicin (two-thirds of the minimum expected allicin yield of a clove of fresh garlic).

Heavy Metal Contamination: Must not exceed California Prop 65 levels for lead contamination in a recommended daily serving and, in no event, exceed 2 mcg of lead in a recommended daily serving. (The State of California has established its own strict standards for lead, including 0.5 micrograms of lead per serving per day for foods and most supplements—although this is raised to 1.5 micrograms per daily serving for calcium supplements. Products sold in California that exceed these levels are required to bear warning labels.)

Contain less than 0.3 parts per million (or micrograms per gram of dried root) of cadmium (World Health Organization proposed guidelines).

Meet recommended USP parameters for disintegration for vitamin supplements (excluding capsule, enteric-coated, chewable, and time-release products).

Meet all FDA labeling requirements.

Milk Thistle

Testing Method: Milk thistle products were tested for their total silymarin content (specifically dehydrosilybinin, isosilybinin A and B, silybinin A and B, silychristin and silydianin). All products were first analyzed in an independent laboratory for the silymarin constituents using an HPLC (High Performance Liquid Chromatography) assay. This HPLC method was developed by the Institute for Nutraceutical Advancement's (INA) Method Validation Program (MVP) to specifically test for the presence for these substances. Products not passing this initial assay were tested in a second independent laboratory utilizing a UV assay.*

Analyses for lead were made using Inductively Coupled Plasma/ Mass Spectroscopy (ICP/MS).

Disintegration of nonchewable, noncapsule, nonenteric-coated, and non-time-release formulations was analyzed utilizing USP (United States Pharmacopeia) <2040> recommendations entitled "Disintegration and Dissolution of Nutritional Supplements."

The identities of the products were not disclosed to the laboratories performing the testing.

Passing Score: To achieve a "Pass" in the testing, a product had to meet the following criteria:

Meet all FDA requirements, including listing the following information in its labeling:

Proper plant name (Milk thistle; Silybum marianum; or *Silybum marianum* (L.) Gaertn.);

Part of the plant used (seed/fruit);

Form of milk thistle used (e.g., seed powder, extract, or tincture);

Amount of milk thistle or silymarin per pill or dose in grams (g) or milligrams (mg) [1 gram = 1,000 milligrams]

Meet its label claim for total silymarin content, with a minimum of 1.5% silymarin for seed powder preparations and 70% silymarin for dry extract preparations (wt/wt). Total silymarin was calculated as the sum of dehydrosilybinin, isosilybinin A and B, silybinin A and B, silychristin and silydianin.

Not exceed California's Prop 65 levels for lead contamination in a recommended daily serving and, in no event, exceed 2 mcg of lead in a recommended daily serving.

Meet recommended USP parameters for disintegration for vitamin supplements (excluding capsule, enteric-coated, chewable, and time-release products).

A "Pass" was based on meeting the above criteria in either the first or second rounds of testing.

*It is of scientific interest that results from the HPLC testing uniformly showed lower levels of silymarin than the UV testing. This is due to greater specificity of the HPLC silymarin method. The UV method, however, remains a common method of testing. ConsumerLab.com recommends that future clinical and scientific investigations of milk thistle include HPLC analyses in order to better characterize its active silymarin constituents, develop more uniform standardization, and more accurately determine optimum dosage.

Seed Oils with Omega-6 and -3 Fatty Acids

Testing Methods: Omega-3 and 6 vegetable oil products were tested for amounts of ALA, GLA and other fatty acids as well as for high peroxide levels (which indicate spoilage). All products were analyzed for their ALA, GLA, and other fatty acid components by gas chromatography utilizing a modified AOAC (Association of Official Analytical Chemists, International) Official Method 991.39. Products not passing this initial assay were tested in a second independent laboratory utilizing modified AOCS methods for fatty acid determination. Peroxide values were analyzed using AOCS (American Oil Chemists Society) Methods CD 8-53 & 12-57.

The identities of the products were not disclosed to the laboratories performing the testing.

Passing Score: A product passed if it met the following criteria:
100% of label claims for ALA, GLA, and other claimed fatty acids not to exceed 150% of claimed amount;

A minimum percentage (% wt/wt) of ALA and GLA as listed below for the individual oils types:

Flaxseed oil—min. 40% ALA
Borage oil—min. 20% GLA
Black currant oil— min.12% ALA, 15% GLA
Evening Primrose Oil—min. 7% GLA
A peroxide value of no more than 10 meq/kg

A "Pass" was based on meeting the above criteria in either the first or second rounds of testing.

St. John's Wort

Testing Methods: St. John's wort products were tested for their amount of total hypericin, total hyperforin (if claimed) and potential contamination with lead and cadmium and their ability to disintegrate (break apart) properly. All products were analyzed for total hypericin using both the Deutscher Arzneimittel-Codex method (DAC '86 Rev. '91) and a separate high performance liquid chromatography (HPLC) method for hyperforin (Institute for Nutraceutical Advancement (INA)).

Analyses for lead and cadmium were made using Inductively Coupled Plasma/Mass Spectroscopy (ICP/MS) or Atomic Absorption/ Graphite Furnace.

Disintegration of nonchewable, noncapsule, nonenteric-coated, and non-time-release formulations was analyzed utilizing USP (United States Pharmacopeia) <2040> recommendations entitled "Disintegration and Dissolution of Nutritional Supplements."

Any product that did not pass the testing was sent to another independent laboratory to repeat testing for at least one of the criteria on which it did not pass. The identities of the products were not disclosed to the laboratories performing the testing.

ConsumerLab.com may modify or use other appropriate test methods if necessary to test special product formulations.

Passing Score: To achieve a "Pass" in the testing, a product had to meet the following criteria:

Meet its label claims for total hypericin and total hyperforin, with a minimum of 0.3% total hypericins for extracts and 0.1% total hypericins for herb (common industry standard).

Not exceed California Prop 65 levels for lead contamination in a recommended daily serving and, in no event, exceed 2 mcg of lead in a recommended daily serving.

Contain less than 0.3 parts per million (or micrograms per gram) of cadmium for dried raw herb (World Health Organization, Quality Control Methods for Medicinal Plant Material, proposed guidelines, 1998), or less than 0.1 part per million for extracts. The lower concentration standard for extracts reflects the ability to remove heavy metals such as cadmium during the extraction process.

Meet recommended USP parameters for disintegration for dietary supplements (excluding capsule, enteric-coated, chewable, and time-release products).

Product must meet all FDA labeling requirements.

A "Pass" was based on meeting the above criteria in either the first or second rounds of testing.

Valerian

Testing Method: Valerian products were tested for their total valerenic acid content (specifically acetoxyvalerenic acid, hydroxyvalerenic acid, and valerenic acid) and valernal. All products were first analyzed in an independent laboratory for the valerenic acid constituents using an HPLC (High Performance Liquid Chromatography) assay. This HPLC method was developed by the Institute for Nutraceutical Advancement's (INA) Method Validation Program (MVP) to specifically test for the presence for these substances. Products not passing this initial assay were tested in a second independent laboratory utilizing a similar HPLC assay.

Analyses for lead and cadmium were made using Inductively Coupled Plasma/Mass Spectroscopy (ICP/MS) or Atomic Absorption/Graphite Furnace.

Disintegration of nonchewable, noncapsule, nonenteric-coated, and non-time-release formulations was analyzed utilizing USP (United States Pharmacopeia) <2040> recommendations entitled "Disintegration and Dissolution of Nutritional Supplements."

The identities of the products were not disclosed to the laboratories performing the testing.

Passing Score: To achieve a "Pass" in the testing, a product had to meet the following criteria:

Meet all FDA requirements, including listing the following information in its labeling:

Proper plant name (Valerian; *Valeriana officinalis* L.);

Part of the plant used (root/rhizome);

Form of valerian used (e.g., root powder, extract, or tincture);

Amount of valerian per pill or dose in grams (g) or milligrams (mg) [1 gram = 1,000 milligrams]

Meet its label claim for total valerenic acid content, with a minimum of 0.17% total valerenic acids for root powder (dried herb) preparations. Extracts or tinctures of 3:1 to 6:1 ratios were expected to have minimum total valerenic acids of 0.4%–0.8%, respectively—with 0.4% the minimum if a concentration was not stated on the label. Total valerenic acids were calculated as the sum of acetoxyvalerenic acid, hydroxyvalerenic acid, and valerenic acid. (Note hydroxyvalerenic acid may be a degradation product rather than an inherent marker compound.)

Not exceed California's Prop 65 levels for lead contamination in a recommended daily serving and, in no event, exceed 2 mcg of lead in a recommended daily serving.

Contain less than 0.3 parts per million (or micrograms per gram) of cadmium for dried herb or extract. This is based on the World Health Organization, Quality Control Methods for Medicinal Plant Material, proposed guidelines, 1998). Although this guideline was developed for dried herb, the same standard is applied here to extracts because heavy metals should be removed during the extraction process.

Meet recommended USP parameters for disintegration for vitamin supplements (excluding capsule, enteric coated, chewable and time-release products).

A "Pass" was based on meeting the above criteria in either the first or second rounds of testing.

Vitamin and Mineral Products

B Vitamins

Testing Methods: B vitamin products were tested for amounts of the B vitamins thiamine, (thiamin HCl), total vitamin B-2 (riboflavin and derivatives), total B-3 (niacin and niacinamide), total B-5 (pantothenic acid), total B-6 (pyridoxine HCl and derivatives), folic acid, biotin, and total B-12. The products were also tested for their ability to disintegrate in solution (excluding chewable and time-release products).

Products were analyzed for B vitamin elements using the USP (United States Pharmacopoeia) 24 and AOAC methods for Water-soluble Vitamin Tablets in independent laboratories.

Disintegration of nonchewable and non-time-release formulations was analyzed utilizing USP (United States Pharmacopoeia) <2040> recommendations entitled "Disintegration and Dissolution of Nutritional Supplements."

All testing was conducted by independent laboratories to which the identities of the products were not disclosed.

Passing Score: To pass, a product had to meet the following criteria:

Contain at least 100% and no more than 150% of its claimed amount of the B vitamins included in the testing.

Meet recommended USP parameters for disintegration for vitamin supplements (excluding chewable and time-release products).

Clearly and accurately state the amount of minerals and vitamins (oil- and water-soluble) expected to be in the product.

A product that passed the above criteria but exceeds any Tolerable Upper Intake Level (UL) established by the Institute of Medicine of the National Academies for any ingredients for the product's intended population was indicated with an explanatory footnote of precautions.

A "Pass" was based on meeting the above criteria in either the first or second rounds of testing. Retesting was performed in a second independent laboratory.

Chromium

Testing Method: Each product was tested for its amount of chromium. Analysis included identification of potential contamination with hexavalent chromium. The products were also tested for their amounts of bitter orange (sour orange, *Citrus aurantium* L.), if claimed, and caffeine, if claimed. Products were also tested for their ability to disintegrate in solution (excluding capsules, chewable, and time-release products). The following testing methods were employed.

Bitter orange products were quantitatively analyzed for synephrine-type alkaloids (synephrine, hordenine, N-methyl tyramine, octopamine, tyramine) by High Performance Liquid Chromatography (HPLC), Capillary Electrophoresis (CE), and screened by Gas Chromatography with Mass Spectral Detection (GC-MS).

Chromium products were analyzed using an Inductively Coupled Plasma-Mass Spectroscopy (ICP-MS) for total chromium and Ion Chromatography (EPA method 3060A/7199) for hexavalent chromium (chromium VI).

In addition, any product claiming to contain bitter orange or a stimulant blend was screened for stimulants and related compounds by Gas Chromatography. Confirmation of any detected banned substances was made by GC-mass spectroscopy. Products were quantitatively analyzed for xanthine alkaloids (caffeine, theophylline, and theobromine) by HPLC.

Disintegration of noncapsule, nonchewable, and non-time-release formulations was analyzed utilizing USP (United States Pharmacopeia) <2040> recommendations entitled "Disintegration and Dissolution of Nutritional Supplements."

Lead was analyzed by ICP-MS.

Products not having passing levels of key ingredients or contaminants were then retested in a another independent laboratory using similar methods and instrumentation. The identities of the products were not disclosed to the laboratories performing the testing.

Passing Score: To achieve a "Pass" in the testing, a product had to meet the following criteria:

Bitter Orange/Stimulant Blend Products had to contain a minimum of 100% and no more than 135% of label claim for synephrine and contain other bitter orange alkaloids (hordenine, N-methyl tyramine, octopamine, tyramine) in appropriate levels 4:1. Dry extracts without label claim should have no less than 1% synephrine and no more than 6% (%wt/wt of peel extract) and contain other bitter orange alkaloids (hordenine, N-methyl tyramine, octopamine, tyramine) in appropriate levels 4:1.

Contain 100% and no more than 120% of label claim for xanthine alkaloids (as caffeine, theophylline, and theobromine).

These products also could contain no detectable amounts of stimulants if the products did not claim to contain caffeine, stimulants or related ingredients.

Chromium Products had to contain a minimum of 100% and no more than 120% of the label claim for total chromium.

They also had to contain less than 0.1% of hexavalent chromium (chromium VI) by %wt/wt of total chromium.

All Products could not exceed California Prop 65 levels for lead contamination in a recommended daily serving and, in no event, exceed 2 mcg of lead in a recommended daily serving. (The State of California has established its own strict standards for lead, including 0.5 micrograms of lead per serving per day for foods and most supplements. Products sold in California that exceed these levels are required to bear warning labels.)

They also had to meet recommended USP parameters for disintegration for nutritional supplements (excluding capsule, chewable, and time-release products).

Meet all FDA labeling requirements.

A "Pass" was based on passing each criterion in any one of the analyses.

Iron

Testing Method: Products were tested for their amount of iron, disintegration, and potential contamination with lead. Analyses for iron and lead were first performed using an atomic absorption/flame method and ICP-MS (Inductively Coupled Plasma-Mass Spectroscopy) in an independent laboratory. Products not having passing levels of iron or lead were then retested for the specific metal using an atomic absorption/flame and atomic absorption/graphite furnace methods respectively in a second independent laboratory. Disintegration of nonchewable and non-time-release formulations was analyzed utilizing USP (United States Pharmacopeia) <2040> recommendations entitled "Disintegration and Dissolution of Nutritional Supplements."

The identities of the products were not disclosed to the laboratories performing the testing.

Passing Score: To achieve a "Pass" in the testing, a product had to meet the following criteria:

Provide all of the following information in its labeling (as required by the FDA):

The form and amount of iron and all other vitamins, minerals, and other primary ingredients listed;

If the product contained herbs:

The proper plant name;

The part of the plant used (e.g., root/rhizome);

The form of herb used (e.g., root powder, extract, or tincture);

The amount of herb per pill or dose in grams (g) or milligrams (mg) [1 gram = 1,000 milligrams]

Contain 100% of its labeled amount of elemental iron and no more than 125% of this amount.

Meet recommended USP parameters for disintegration of nutritional supplements (excluding chewable and time-release products).

Contain less than 0.5 micrograms of lead per the greater of either (a) 18 mg of elemental iron or (b) the product's maximum suggested daily serving. (Note: The State of California Proposition 65 law requires products exceeding 0.5 mg of lead per suggested daily serving to bear a warning label.)

Provide proper packaging of pills to avoid accidental poisoning in children (child resistant bottle caps, blister packaging, etc.) for products containing 30 mg or more of iron per pill.

A "Pass" was based on passing each criterion in any one of the analyses.

Magnesium

Testing Methods: Products were tested for the ability to disintegrate, the amount of magnesium, and the amount of lead.

Analyses for magnesium and lead were first performed using an ICP-MS (Inductively Coupled Plasma-Mass Spectroscopy) method in an independent laboratory. Products not having passing levels of magnesium or lead were then retested in a second independent laboratory using the similar methods and instrumentation. The identities of the products were not disclosed to the laboratories performing the testing.

Disintegration of nonchewable, noncapsule, nonenteric-coated, and non-time-release formulations was analyzed utilizing USP (United States Pharmacopeia) <2040> recommendations entitled "Disintegration and Dissolution of Nutritional Supplements."

Passing Score: To pass testing, a product had to meet the following criteria:

Have a minimum of 100% of its labeled amount of elemental magnesium and a maximum of 125% of this amount.

Meet purity standards for lead contamination: less than 0.5 micrograms per daily serving in magnesium-only products (California, Proposition 65) or less than 1.5 micrograms per daily serving in magnesium products also containing 1000 mg of elemental calcium.

Meet recommended USP parameters for disintegration for vitamin supplements (excluding capsule, enteric-coated, chewable, and time-release products).

A product passed if it passed each criterion in any one of the analyses.

Multivitamin/Multimineral Supplements

Testing Methods: As described below, products were tested for their amount of selected index elements (see below), their ability to disintegrate in solution (excluding chewable and time-release products), and lead contamination.

Each product was tested for at least one index element in each category shown. The first element within each category was selected unless not claimed in the product, in which case, the next claimed element was selected.

Oil-soluble vitamins

Vitamin A (levels of beta-carotene and retinol (retinyl acetate or palmitate) evaluated independently)

Vitamin E (natural and synthetic forms)

Vitamin D

Water-soluble vitamins

Folic acid (folate)

Vitamin C (ascorbic acid)
B vitamins
    Niacin
    Pyridoxine
    Riboflavin
Minerals
Calcium
Iron
Zinc
Magnesium
Manganese

Products were analyzed for their vitamin and mineral index elements using the USP (United States Pharmacopeia) methods for oil- and water-soluble vitamins and mineral tablets in an independent laboratory.

Disintegration of nonchewable and non-time-release formulations was analyzed utilizing USP (United States Pharmacopeia) <2040> recommendations entitled "Disintegration and Dissolution of Nutritional Supplements."

Analyses for lead were performed using an atomic absorption/graphite furnace method or ICP-MS (Inductively Coupled Plasma-Mass Spectroscopy).

All testing was conducted in independent laboratories, in which the identities of the products were not disclosed.

Passing Score: To achieve a "Pass" in the testing, a product had to meet the following criteria:

Contain at least 100% and no more than 150% of its claimed amount of the index elements. Any product claiming vitamin A had to meet its claimed amount for total vitamin A (beta-carotene and retinol combined) as well as meet any claimed ratio of beta-carotene to total vitamin A.

Meet recommended USP parameters for disintegration for supplements (excluding chewable and time-release products). These parameters include a limit of 30 minutes for uncoated and film-coated vitamin-mineral tablets and a limit of 45 minutes for plain coated vitamin-mineral tablets.

Meet the State of California's Prop 65 limits for lead in supplements: 0.5 mcg of lead per daily serving with an additional allowance of 1.0 mcg for supplements containing 1,000 mg/day or more of elemental calcium and 0.5 mcg for supplements containing specific other minerals. For supplements not marketed for use by children, ConsumerLab.com provides an additional allowance of 0.5

mcg if containing 250 to 499 mg/day of elemental calcium or 1.0 mcg if containing 500 to 999 mg/day of elemental calcium and an allowance of 0.5 mcg for if containing one herb or 1.0 mcg for two or more herbs.

Meet all FDA labeling requirements.

For a product to fail, confirmation of a failing result was required on at least one of the criteria through repeat testing in a second independent laboratory.

Potassium

Testing Methods: Products were tested for the ability to disintegrate, the amount of potassium, and the amount of lead. Analyses for potassium and lead were first performed using an atomic absorption/graphite furnace method and ICP-MS (Inductively Coupled Plasma-Mass Spectroscopy) in an independent laboratory. Products not having passing levels of potassium or lead were then retested in a second independent laboratory using the similar methods and instrumentation. The identities of the products were not disclosed to the laboratories performing the testing.

Disintegration of nonchewable, noncapsule, nonenteric-coated, and non-time-release formulations was analyzed utilizing USP (United States Pharmacopeia) <2040> recommendations entitled "Disintegration and Dissolution of Nutritional Supplements."

Passing Score: To pass testing, a product had to meet the following criteria:

Have a minimum of 100% of its labeled amount of elemental potassium and a maximum of 125% of this amount.

Contain less than 0.5 micrograms of lead per daily serving—corresponding to the limit established for potassium-only products in the State of California's Proposition 65.

Meet recommended USP parameters for disintegration for vitamin/mineral supplements (excluding capsule, enteric-coated, chewable, and time-release products).

A product passed if it passed each criterion in any one of the analyses.

Vitamin C

Testing Method: Vitamin C products were tested for their amount of vitamin C and their ability to disintegrate in solution (excluding capsules, chewable, and time-release products). All products were first analyzed utilizing a HPLC (High Performance Liquid Chromatography) assay in an independent laboratory. Products not passing this initial assay were tested in a second independent laboratory using the AOAC (Association of Official Analytical Chemists) Official Method 43.064—Microfluorometric Method for Quantitation of Vitamin C (ascorbic acid) in an independent laboratory. Disintegration of noncapsule, nonchewable, and non-time-release formulations was analyzed utilizing USP (United States Pharmacopeia) <2040> recommendations entitled "Disintegration and Dissolution of Nutritional Supplements." The identities of the products were not disclosed to the laboratories performing the testing.

Passing Score: To achieve a "Pass" in the testing, a product had to first contain at least 100% and no more than 120% of its claimed amount of vitamin C and, second, meet recommended USP parameters for disintegration for vitamin supplements (excluding capsules, chewable, and time-release products). The amount of vitamin C in the product also had to be clearly and accurately stated in the labeling. A pass was based on meeting the criteria for both vitamin C quantity and, if applicable, disintegration, in either the first or second rounds of testing.

Vitamin E

Testing Method: Vitamin E products were tested for their identity and amount of vitamin E. All products were first analyzed for various vitamin E forms including mixed tocopherols using a HPLC (High Performance Liquid Chromatography) Tocopherol assay in an independent laboratory. Products not passing this initial assay were tested in a second independent laboratory utilizing a similar HPLC assay (USP 26)(United States Pharmacopeia). Products claiming to contain natural forms of vitamin E were analyzed by optical rotation also utilizing the USP 26 assay and a HPLC chiral separation. Disintegration of nonchewable and non-time-release formulations was analyzed utilizing USP (United States Pharmacopeia) <2040> recommendations entitled "Disintegration and Dissolution of Nutritional Supplements."

The identities of the products were not disclosed to the laboratories performing the testing.

Passing Score: To achieve a "Pass" in the testing, a product had to meet the following criteria:

Contain at least 100% and no more than 120% of its claimed amount of its labeled form of vitamin E.

If claimed to contain natural vitamin E, the product had to meet recommended USP parameters for the specific rotation for natural vitamin E supplements (not less than +24°) and contain no synthetic vitamin E (d-alpha-tocopheryl acid succinate and acetate are stabilized forms of natural vitamin E).

Clearly and accurately state the amount of vitamin E in the labeling.

Meet recommended USP parameters for disintegration of nutritional supplements (excluding chewable and time-release products).

A "Pass" was based on passing each criterion in any one of the analyses.

Zinc

Testing Methods: Zinc products were tested for their elemental zinc content, potential contamination with lead, and their ability to disintegrate (break apart) properly. Analyses for zinc and lead were made using Inductively Coupled Plasma/Mass Spectroscopy (ICP/MS) or Atomic Absorption/Graphite Furnace.

Disintegration of nonchewable, noncapsule, nonenteric-coated, and non-time-release formulations were analyzed utilizing USP (United States Pharmacopeia) <2040> recommendations entitled "Disintegration and Dissolution of Nutritional Supplements."

Any product that did not pass the testing was sent to another independent laboratory to repeat testing for at least one of the criteria on which it did not pass. The identities of the products were not disclosed to the laboratories performing the testing.

Passing Score: To achieve a "Pass" in the testing, a product had to meet the following criteria:

Have a minimum of 100% of its labeled amount of elemental zinc and a maximum of 150% of this amount.

Not exceed California Prop 65 levels for lead contamination in a recommended daily serving and, in no event, exceed 2 mcg of lead in a recommended daily serving.

Meet recommended USP parameters for disintegration for vitamin supplements (excluding capsule, enteric-coated, chewable, and time-release products).

Product must meet all FDA labeling requirements.

A "Pass" was based on meeting the above criteria in either the first or second rounds of testing.

Special Ingredients

Alpha-Lipoic Acid

Testing Method: Products containing alpha-lipoic acid were first analyzed by High Performance Liquid Chromatography (HPLC). Products that did not pass this initial test were similarly reanalyzed in a second independent laboratory.

Analyses for lead were made using Inductively Coupled Plasma/ Mass Spectroscopy (ICP/MS).

Disintegration of non-chewable, non-capsule, non-enteric-coated, and non-time-release formulations were analyzed utilizing USP (United States Pharmacopeia) <2040> recommendations entitled "Disintegration and Dissolution of Nutritional Supplements."

ConsumerLab.com may modify or use other appropriate test methods if necessary to test special product formulations. Analyses were conducted in independent laboratories to which the brand identities of the products were not disclosed. Any product not passing an initial analysis was retested in a second independent laboratory on at least one of the criteria on which it did not initially pass.

Passing Score: To pass testing, a product must meet the following criteria:

Contain at least 100%, and not more than 150%, of claimed amount of alpha-lipoic acid.

Meet recommended USP parameters for disintegration for vitamin supplements (excluding capsule, enteric-coated, chewable, and time-release products).

Meet all FDA labeling requirements.

Not exceed California's Prop 65 levels for lead contamination in a recommended daily serving and, in no event, exceed 2 mcg of lead in a recommended daily serving.

A product passed if it passed each applicable criterion in any one of the analyses.

CLA (Conjugated Linoleic Acid)

Testing Methods: The CLA weight loss products were analyzed for their CLA isomer fatty acid components by Gas Chromatography

(GC) utilizing a modified AOAC method (Association of Official Analytical Chemists, International; Official Method 991.39).

Disintegration of noncapsule, nonchewable, and non-time-release formulations was analyzed utilizing USP (United States Pharmacopeia) <2040> recommendations entitled "Disintegration and Dissolution of Nutritional Supplements."

Products not having passing levels of key ingredients or contaminants were then retested in a second independent laboratory using similar methods and instrumentation. The identities of the products were not disclosed to the laboratories performing the testing.

Passing Score: To achieve a "Pass" in the testing, a product had to meet the following criteria:

Contain a minimum of 100% of its labeled amount and a maximum of 135% of total CLA and specified CLA isomer ratios.

Not exceed California Prop 65 levels for lead contamination in a recommended daily serving and, in no event, exceed 2 mcg of lead in a recommended daily serving. (The State of California has established its own strict standards for lead, including 0.5 micrograms of lead per serving per day for foods and most supplements. Products sold in California that exceed these levels are required to bear warning labels.)

Meet recommended USP parameters for disintegration for nutritional supplements (excluding capsule, chewable and time-release products).

Meet all FDA labeling requirements.

A product passed if it passed each criterion in any one of the analyses.

CoQ10 (Coenzyme Q10)

Testing Method: Products were tested for their claimed amount of CoQ10. Analysis for CoQ10 was performed using an HPLC method (USP method) in an independent laboratory. Products not having passing levels of CoQ10 were then retested in a second independent laboratory using the same HPLC method.

Disintegration of nonchewable, noncapsule, nonenteric-coated, and non-time-release formulations were analyzed utilizing USP (United States Pharmacopeia) <2040> recommendations entitled "Disintegration and Dissolution of Nutritional Supplements."

Analyses were conducted in independent laboratories to which the brand identities of the products were not disclosed. Any product not passing an initial analysis was retested in a second independent laboratory on at least one of the criteria on which it did not initially pass.

Passing Score: To pass testing, a product had to meet the following criteria:

Contain at least 100% of its labeled amount of CoQ10 and no more than 150% of this amount.

Meet recommended USP parameters for disintegration for vitamin supplements (excluding capsule, enteric-coated, chewable, and time-release products).

Meet all FDA labeling requirements.

A product passed if it passed each applicable criterion in any one of the analyses.

DHEA

Testing Method: Products were tested for their ability to disintegrate, claimed amount of DHEA, and for potential contamination with various anabolic agents. Analysis for DHEA was performed using by High Performance Liquid Chromatography (HPLC) method in an independent laboratory. Products not having passing levels of DHEA were then retested in a second independent laboratory using an HPLC method. Screening for anabolic agents and related substances (see list below) was performed by Gas Chromatography and confirmed with Mass Spectrometry.

Anabolic agents and related substances for which products were tested

androstenediol and analogs	nandrolone and analogs
androstenedione and analogs	19-norandrostenediol
clenbuterol	19-norandrostenedione
clostebol	norethandrolone
fenoterol	oxandrolone
fluoxymesterone	oxymesterone
mesterolone	oxymetholone
metandienone	stanozolol
metenolone (metheneolone)	testosterone and various salts
methandriol	trenbolone
methyltestosterone	

Disintegration of nonchewable, noncapsule, and non-time-release formulations was analyzed utilizing USP (United States Pharmacopeia) <2040> recommendations entitled "Disintegration and Dissolution of Nutritional Supplements." Any product that did not pass the disintegration testing was sent to another independent laboratory in which the same test was repeated.

The identities of the products were not disclosed to the laboratories performing the testing.

Passing Score: To pass testing, a product had to meet the following criteria:

Have a minimum of 100% of its labeled amount of DHEA and a maximum of 125% of this amount.

Meet recommended USP parameters for disintegration for dietary supplements (excluding capsule, chewable, and time-release products).

Contain less than 0.1% androstenedione (a manufacturing by-product of synthetic DHEA) and no other confirmed anabolic substance or related substance listed above.

A product passed if it passed each criterion in any one of the analyses.

Melatonin

Testing Method: Analysis for melatonin and lead was performed using an HPLC method and ICP-MS (Inductively Coupled Plasma-Mass Spectroscopy) in an independent laboratory. Products not having passing levels of melatonin or lead were then retested in a second independent laboratory using comparable HPLC and ICP-MS methods.

Disintegration of non-chewable, non-capsule, and non-time-release formulations was analyzed utilizing USP (United States Pharmacopeia) <2040> recommendations entitled "Disintegration and Dissolution of Nutritional Supplements." Any product that did not pass the disintegration testing was sent to another independent laboratory in which the same test was repeated.

The identities of the products were not disclosed to the laboratories performing the testing.

Passing Score: To pass testing, a product must meet the following criteria:

Contain a minimum of 100% of its labeled amount of melatonin and not exceed 135% of this amount.

Meet recommended USP parameters for disintegration for vitamin supplements (excluding capsule, enteric-coated, chewable, and time-release products).

Contain less than 0.5 micrograms of lead per daily serving.

Meet FDA labeling requirements.

A "Pass" was based on meeting the above criteria in either the first or second rounds of testing.

Omega-3 Fatty Acids (DHA & EPA, Fish/Marine) Oils

Testing Method: Omega-3 marine oil products were tested for the amounts of their EPA and DHA omega-3 fatty acids, peroxide value, anisidine value, TOTOX and potential contamination with mercury and PCB. All products were assessed for their EPA and DHA components by gas chromatography utilizing a modified AOAC method (Association of Official Analytical Chemists, International; Official Method 991.39); for peroxide value using AOCS method (American Oil Chemists Society; Method CD 8-53 or similar); for anisidine value using AOCS method (Method CD 18-90 or similar); for mercury using a Cold Vapor Atomic Absorption method; and for PCBs using High Resolution Gas Chromatography coupled with High Resolution Mass Spectrometry (EPA Method 1668A) in independent laboratories. Products not passing the initial assay for EPA and DHA, peroxide value, anisidine value, TOTOX, and mercury were tested in another independent laboratory utilizing a similar method.

Several products tested through the Voluntary Certification Program were also tested, at the special request of their manufacturers, for dioxin contamination. Dioxin testing was performed using EPA method 1663B. The identities of the products were not disclosed to the laboratories performing the testing.

Passing Score: To achieve a "Pass" in the testing a product must meet the following criteria:

Contain 100% and not exceed 150% of the claimed amounts of omega-3 fatty acids, EPA and DHA;

Have a peroxide value (PV) of no more than 5 meq/kg, an anisidine value (AV) of no more than 20, and a TOTOX value of no more than 26 (calculated as (2 x PV) + AV) (CRN Monograph Recomendation);

Contain less than 0.1 ppm of mercury (CRN Monograph Recomendation);

Contain less than 0.09 mg/kg (ppm) of Total PCBs (sum of four non-ortho PCBs and eight mono-ortho PCBs). (CRN Monograph Recomendation);

If tested for dioxins (sum of 17 individual dioxin congeners), contain no more than 2 TEF/g (expressed in World Health Organization (WHO) toxic equivalents as WHO-toxic equivalent factors (TEFs). (CRN Monograph Recomendation)

A "Pass" was based on meeting the above criteria in either the first or second rounds of testing.

Probiotics

Testing Methods: Products were tested for their ability to disintegrate, amount of anaerobic lactic acid fermenting microorganisms, and contamination with other microbes. Analysis for the enumeration of *L. acidophilus* and other freeze-dried lactic acid microorganisms was performed using procedures as outlined in *The Standard Methods for the Examination of Dairy Products* (16th ed.), using a modified De Man Rogosa and Sharpe agar (MRS) to which L-cysteine HCl was added and another media, a Reinforced Clostridial agar (Oxoid). Products not having passing levels of anaerobic microorganisms were then retested in a second independent laboratory using comparable methods.

Analyses for microbial contaminants were made using methods from the FDA's *Bacteriological Analytical Manual* (BAM) and included testing for *Escherichia coli, Salmonella* spp. *Staphylococcus aureus, Pseudomonas aeruginosa,* and other enteric bacteria including *Klebsiella, Enterobacter, Proteus, Citrobacter, Aerobacter, Providencia,* and *Serratia*. Testing also included analyses for total yeast and mold.

Disintegration of nonchewable and noncapsule formulations was analyzed utilizing USP (United States Pharmacopeia) <2040> recommendations entitled "Disintegration and Dissolution of Nutritional Supplements" and 701 recommendations (enteric coated). Any product that did not pass the disintegration testing was sent to another independent laboratory in which the same test was repeated. The identities of the products were not disclosed to the laboratories performing the testing.

Passing Score: To pass testing, a product had to meet the following criteria:

Have a minimum of 100% of its labeled amount of total anaerobic microorganisms or meet 1 billion microorganisms per maximum recommended daily serving, whichever is greater.

Meet recommended USP parameters for disintegration for enteric-coated tablets and dietary supplements (excluding capsule and chewable products).

Test negative for *Escherichia coli, Salmonella* spp., *Staphylococcus aureus*, and *Pseudomonas aeruginosa* (as required by the FDA). In addition, contain less than 100 CFU per gram for total coliform and total yeast/mold.

A product passed if it passed each criterion in any one of the analyses.

SAMe

Testing Methods: SAMe products were tested for their levels of the S-adenosyl-methionine (SAMe). As the molecule can break down under certain circumstances, products were also tested for levels of breakdown products. Testing was first conducted in an independent laboratory using high performance liquid chromatography (HPLC). Products that did not pass these two tests were reanalyzed using another HPLC method in a second independent laboratory.

Disintegration of enteric-coated formulations were analyzed utilizing USP (United States Pharmacopeia) <701> recommendations.

Analyses were conducted in independent laboratories to which the brand identities of the products were not disclosed. Any product not passing an initial analysis was retested in a second independent laboratory on at least one of the criteria on which it did not initially pass.

Passing Score: To pass testing, a product had to meet the following criteria:

Contain its claimed weight of SAMe and no more than 110% of that weight. The amount of "free" SAMe (i.e., not including stabilizing compounds) had to be clearly and accurately stated in the label. Total SAMe degradation products (combined levels of adenine, S-adenosyl-L-homocysteine [SAH], and methylthioadenosine [MTA]) could not exceed 10% of the claimed weight of "free" SAMe.

Meet recommended USP parameters for disintegration for enteric-coated tablets and dietary supplements (excluding capsule and chewable products).

Meet all FDA labeling requirements.

A product passed if it passed each applicable criterion in any one of the analyses.

Nutrition Bars, Powders, and Drinks

Nutrition Bars: High-Protein, Low-Carb-Diet, Energy, and Meal-Replacement

Testing Methods: Nutrition bar products were tested for their total calories, total fat, poly- and monounsaturated fat, saturated fat, cholesterol, protein, total carbohydrates, total sugars, sugar alcohols, and sodium content. All products were first analyzed for their specific nutritional components using AOAC (Association of Official Analytical Chemists, International) methods in an independent laboratory. Products not passing this initial assay for any specific nutrient were tested in a second independent laboratory utilizing similar AOAC methods.

The identities of the products were not disclosed to the laboratories performing the testing.

Passing Score: To achieve a "Pass" in the testing, a product had to meet the following criteria:

Specify the amount of all nutrients in the product that are required by the FDA to be stated in the Nutrition Facts panel for foods or in the Supplement Facts panel for dietary supplements.

Meet its label claims within a specified range for each nutritional component as indicated below:

Total Fat (within 1 gram or 10% above claim, whichever is greater)

Saturated Fat (within 0.5 gram or 10% above claim, whichever is greater)

Cholesterol (within 2 mg or 10% above claim, whichever is greater)

Sodium (within 100 mg or 10% above claim, whichever is greater)

Protein (within +/− 20% of claim)

Total Carbohydrates (within +/− 5 grams of claim)

Total Sugars (within 1 gram or 10% above claim, whichever is greater)

Total Calories (within +/− 20% of claim)

A "Pass" was based on meeting the above criteria in either the first or second rounds of testing.

Nutrition Powders, Shakes and Drinks: Protein, Diet, General Nutrition, and Meal Replacements

Testing Methods: Nutrition powder and drinks products were tested for their total calories, total fat, poly- and monounsaturated fat, saturated fat, cholesterol, protein, total carbohydrates, total sugars and sodium content. All products were first analyzed for their specific nutritional components using AOAC (Association of Official Analytical Chemists, International) methods in an independent laboratory. Products not passing this initial assay for any specific nutrient were tested in a second independent laboratory utilizing similar AOAC methods.

The identities of the products were not disclosed to the laboratories performing the testing.

Passing Score: To achieve a "Pass" in the testing, a product had to meet the following criteria:

Specify the amount of all nutrients in the product as required by the FDA and be appropriately classified as a food or dietary supplement.

Meet its label claims within a specified range for each nutritional component as indicated below:

Total Fat (within 1 gram or 15% of claim, whichever is greater; or, if claiming zero total fat, no more than 0.5 gram/serving);

Saturated Fat (within 0.5 gram/serving or 15% above claim, whichever is greater);

Cholesterol (within 4 mg/serving or 15% above claim, whichever is greater; or, if claiming zero cholesterol, no more than 2 mg/serving);

Sodium (within 50 mg/serving or 15% above claim, whichever is greater; or, if claiming zero sodium, no more than 5 mg/serving);

Protein (within 1 gram/serving or 15% of claim, whichever is greater);

Total Carbohydrates (within 5 gram/serving or 15% of claim, whichever is greater; or, if claiming zero to 3g/serving of carbohydrates, within 1g of claim);

Total Sugars (within 1 gram/serving or 15% above claim, whichever is greater; or, if claiming zero sugar, within 0.5 gram/serving of claim)

Total Calories (within +/− 20% of claim)

A "Pass" was based on meeting the above criteria in either the first or second rounds of testing.

Banned Substances

Testing Methods: Screening involves one or more analytic methods, for example, HPLC or GC, and includes spiking and recovery of certain compounds to insure proper extraction. Confirmation of any detected banned substances is made by mass spectroscopy.

Passing Score: To pass, a product must contain no confirmed Banned Substance at a "zero-tolerance level"—defined by the recovery rate of a substance as well as its limit of detection in a given matrix.

Online Resources

ConsumerLab.com

This Web site offers online subscribers access to product reviews including those in this book as well as new reviews and updates. It also provides recent and archived recalls and warnings and a comprehensive encyclopedia of natural products and drug interactions. Readers will find free general information as well as subscription-only content. Readers can also sign up for a free newsletter alerting them when new reviews and articles are posted. www.consumerlab.com

Government Resources

FDA Enforcement Report Index

This Web site is published weekly by the FDA. It contains information on actions taken in connection with agency regulatory activities. http://www.fda.gov/opacom/Enforce.html

Food and Nutrition Board of the Institute of Medicine

(National Academy of Sciences)
The Food and Nutrition Board convenes experts to develop nutritional recommendations. Its reports, which are available free online or for purchase in print, provide the scientific basis for the recommendations. Of particular importance are its reports on Dietary Reference Intakes, which establish the recommended daily amounts and upper limits for vitamins and minerals. http://www.iom.edu/CMS/3788.aspx

MedWatch: Reporting adverse events

MedWatch allows both health care professionals and consumers to report serious problems that they suspect are associated with drugs and medical devices. Reporting can be done online, by phone, or by submitting the MedWatch 3500 form by mail or fax. http://www.fda.gov/medwatch/how.htm

More Brand Information

Here, we've provided manufacturer and distributor Web addresses and phone numbers for each brand listed in the reviews. Some brands include additional product information from the manufacturer or distributor; that product information is considered advertising. This information was current when the book went to press but may change anytime.

AARP
Memory, Multivitamins/ Multiminerals
AARP
www.aarppharmacy.com
800-456-2277

Aboca
Valerian
Aboca S.p.A
www.aboca.us
877-226-2248

AccuTech, LLC
Cholesterol Lowering
AccuTech, LLC
accutech-llc.com
800-749-9910

Action Labs
Ginseng
Nutraceutical Corp.
www.nutraceutical.com
800-579-4665

Advocare
Joint Care, Omega-3, Probiotics
Advocare International
www.advocare.com
800-348-7806

Akyma
B Vitamins
Akyma Pharmacticals LLC
www.akyma.com
866-525-7270

Albi Imports, Ltd.
Cholesterol Lowering
Albi Imports, Ltd.
www.albi-imports.com
800-663-0628

Allergy Research Group
CoQ10, Omega-3, Seed Oils
Allergy Research Group
www.allergyresearchgroup.com
800-545-9960

Allmax
CLA
Allmax Nutrition Inc.
www.allmaxnutrition.com
800-409-7111

Alluna
Valerian
Enzymetic Therapy, Inc.
www.enzy.com
800-558-7372

More Brand Information

Amerifit Nutrition
Memory
Amerifit Nutrition
www.amerifit.com
800-722-3476

Amino Vital
Banned Substances
Ajinomoto Co., Inc.
www.amino-vital.com
888-264-6673

Andrew Lessman
Alpha-Lipoic Acid, Bone Health
YourVitamins, Inc.
www.procapslabs.com
888-888-2876

ArginMax
Sexual Enhancement
The Daily Wellness Company
www.dailywellness.com
800-988-4869

Arizona Natural
Garlic
ANP Inc.
www.arizonanatural.com
800-255-2823

Ark Naturals
Probiotics (Pets)
Ark Naturals
www.arknaturals.com
800-926-5100

AST
CLA, DHEA
AST Sports Science
www.ast-ss.com
800-627-2788

Atkins
Nutrition Bar, Nutrition Powder
Atkins Nutritionals Inc.
www.atkins.com
800-6-atkins

Balance Bar
Nutrition Bar
Balance Bar Company
www.balance.com

Barefoot Coral
Bone Health
Bently Hubbell International
www.calciumsupreme.com

Barlean's
Seed Oils
Barleans's Organic Oils
http://barleans.com
360-384-0485

Bausch & Lomb Ocuvite
Sight Enhancement
Bausch & Lomb
Pharmaceuticals, Inc.
www.bausch.com
800-227-1427

Baywood Solution
Bone Health, SAMe
Baywood
www.bywd.com
800-481-7169

Berkely & Jensen
(BJ's Warehouse Club)
*Bone Health, Omega-3,
Prostate Health*
BJWC
www.bjs.com

BioChem
Melatonin
Country Life
www.country-life.com
800-645-5768

Bioforce
Valerian
Bioforce USA

Bluebonnet
Cancer Prevention, CoQ10
Bluebonnet Corporation
www.bluebonnetnutrition.com
800-580-8866

Body Fortress
Muscular Enhancement,
Nutrition Powder
U.S. Nutrition
www.bodyfortress.com
800-215-5980

BodyTech
Weight Loss
The Vitamin Shoppe
www.vitaminshoppe.com
800-223-1216

Breeder's Choice
ALA
Breeder's Choice Foods, Inc.
www.breeders-choice.com
800-255-4286

Bronson
Alpha-Lipoic Acid, Joint
Care
Bronson Laboratories
www.bronsononline.com
800-294-5507

Caltrate
Bone Health
Wyeth Consumer Health
www.caltrate.com
888-797-5638

Canadian Sun
Cancer Prevention, Memory,
Seed Oils
Canadian Health Product Ltd.
www.canadiansun.com
800-663-0747

Carb Minders
Nutrition Bar
HealthSmart

Carb Options
Nutrition Bar
Unilever Bestfoods

Carb Solutions
Nutrition Bar
Richardson Labs, Inc.

Carb Watchers
Nutrition Powder
Labrada Nutrition
www.labrada.com
800-832-9948

CarboRite
Nutrition Bar
CarboLite Foods, Inc.

CarbWise
Nutrition Bar
Synergy Plus

Cardiovascular Research
Omega-3, Seed Oils
Cardiovascular Research, Ltd.

Carlson
Cholesterol Lowering, CoQ10,
Omega-3, Potassium, Vitamin E
J.R. Carlson Laboratories
www.carlsonlabs.com
888-234-5656

Centrum
Multivitamins, Sight
Enhancement
Wyeth Consumer Healthcare
www.centrum.com
877-236-8786

More Brand Information

ChildLife Essentials
  Vitamin C
  BioZeal
  www.childlife.net
  800-993-0332

Citracal
  Bone Health
  Mission Pharmacal
  www.citracal.com
  800-531-3333

Clif Luna Bar
  Nutrition Bar
  Clif Bar Inc.
  www.clifbar.com
  800-254-3227

Coral Complex2
  Bone Health
  Coral, Inc.

Coromega
  Omega-3
  ERBL, Inc.
  www.coromega.com
  877-275-3725

CosaminDS
  Joint Care
  Nutramax Laboratories, Inc.
  www.cosamin.com
  800-925-5187

Cosequin
  Joint Care
  Nutramax Laboratories, Inc.
  www.nutramaxlabs.com
  800-925-5187

Country Life
  B Vitamins, Cancer Prevention,
  Joint Care, Milk Thistle, Sight
  Enhancement, Vitamin C
  Country Life
  www.country-life.com
  800-645-5768

Culturelle
  Probiotics
  CAG Functional Foods
  www.culturelle.com
  888-828-4242

CVS
  B Vitamins, Garlic, Ginseng,
  Joint Care, Milk Thistle,
  Omega-3, Sight Enhancement,
  Vitamin C, Vitamin E
  CVS
  www.cvs.com
  800-746-7287

DermCare
  Omega-3
  HAVA Pet Products

Designer Whey
  Nutrition Powder
  Next Proteins
  www.designerwhey.com
  760-431-8152

Designs for Health
  Melatonin, Prostate
  Designs for Health, Inc
  www.designsforhealth.com
  800-847-8302

Dexatrim
  Nutrition Bar
  Chattem, Inc.
  www.dexatrim.com
  800-366-6077

Detour
Nutrition Bar
Next Proteins
www.detourbar.com
760-431-6152

Doctor's Best
Bone Health, CoQ10, Joint Care,
Prostate
Doctor's Best, Inc.
www.doctorsbest.net
800-333-6977

Doctor's Trust
DHEA, Milk Thistle, Potassium,
St. John's Wort
Doctor's Trust Vitamins
www.doctorstrust.com
800-240-6046

Douglas Laboratories
Iron
Douglas Laboratories
www.douglaslabs.com
800-245-4440

Drinkables
Joint Care
Remington Health Products
www.remingtonhealth.com
888-333-4256

Dr. Fuhrman
Multivitamins
DrFuhrman.com, Inc.
www.drfuhrman.com
800-474-9355

Dr. Sears
Nutrition Bar
Sears Labs, Inc.
www.zonelabsinc.com
800-404-8171

Dymatize
Muscular Enhancement,
Sexual Enhancement
Dymatize Enterprises Inc.
www.dymatize.com
800-500-3069

EAS
Muscular Enhancement,
Nutrition Bar, Nutrition Powder
EAS
www.eas.com
800-297-9776

Eckerd
Vitamin C, Zinc
Eckerd Drug Company
www.eckerd.com
800-325-3737

Eclectic Institute
Echinacea, Milk Thistle, Seed
Oils, Valerian
Eclectic Institute Inc.
www.eclecticherb.com
800-332-4372

Eclipse Sport
Muscular Enhancement
Eclipse Sport Supplements
www.eclipsecec.com
800-320-0062

EHP Products
Omega-3
Dist. By EHP Products,Inc.

Emer-gen-C
Vitamin C
Alacer Corp.
www.alacer.com
800-854-0249

Emerita
Menopause
Emerita
www.emerita.com
800-648-8211

More Brand Information

Eniva
  Multivitamins
  Eniva Corporation
  www.eniva.com
  763-795-8870

Enzymatic Therapy
  B Vitamin, Bone Health, DHEA, Omega-3, Probiotics
  Enzymatic Therapy
  www.enzy.com
  800-558-7372

Equaline
  B Vitamin, Potassium
  Albertsons
  www.albertsons.com

Essential Phytosterolins
  Cholesterol Lowering
  Moducare
  www.moducare.com

Estroven
  Bone Health
  Amerifit Nutrition, Inc.
  www.estroven.com
  800-722-3476

Ethical Nutrients
  Vitamin E
  Ethical Nutrients
  www.ethicalnutrients.com
  800-668-8743

Everlast Nutrition
  Muscular Enhancement
  Vitamin Branding Corp.
  www.everlastnutrition.com
  800-737-9055

EZ-Trim
  Chromium
  Scientific Weight Loss Labs
  www.eztrimproducts.com
  866-795-5227

Fairhaven Health
  Multivitamins
  Fairhaven Health, LLC
  www.fairhavenhealth.com
  360-671-0859

Feosol
  Iron
  GlaxoSmithKline Consumer Healthcare
  www.feosol.com
  800-897-7535

Fergon
  Iron
  Bayer
  www.bayercare.com
  800-331-4536

Flintstones
  Bone Health, Multivitamins
  Bayer
  www.bayercare.com
  800-331-4536

Flora Source
  Probiotics
  MBA Company

Floradix
  Iron, Magnesium
  Salus-Haus
  www.florahealth.com
  800-446-2110

Food Lion
  Prostate
  Food Lion LLC
  www.foodlion.com
  800-210-9569

Food Science of Vermont
  Cancer Prevention
  Food Science of Vermont
  www.fslabs.com
  800-874-9444

Futurebiotics
Cancer Prevention, Cholesterol Lowering
Futurebiotics
www.futurebiotics.com
800-645-1721

Gaia Herbs
Menopause, Milk Thistle, St. John's Wort, Valerian
Gaia Herbs, Inc.
www.gaiaherbs.com
888-917-8289

Garden of Life
Omega-3, Probiotics
Garden of Life
http://www.gardenoflifeusa.com/

Garlinase
Garlic
Enzymatic Therapy
www.enzy.com
800-783-2286

Garlique
Garlic
Chattem, Inc.
www.garlique.com

Gary Null
CoQ10, Vitamin C
Gary Null & Associates
www.garynull.com
646-505-4660

GeniSoy
Nutrition Bar, Nutrition Powder
Genisoy Products Co.
www.genisoy.com
888-436-4769

Ginkgo-Go
Memory
Wakunaga of America Co.

Ginkoba
Memory
Alan James Group
www.ginkoba.com
800-451-6688

Ginsana
Ginseng
Alan James Group
www.ginsana.com
800-451-6688

GLC
Joint Care
GLC Direct, LLC
www.glcdirect.com
866-452-3473

GNC
Bone Health, Cancer Prevention, Cholesterol Lowering, CoQ10, Muscular Enhancement, Nutrition Powder, Omega-3, Vitamin E
GNC
www.gnc.com
888-462-2548

Good 'N Natural
Memory
Good 'N Natural Manufacturing Corp.
www.goodnnatural.com

Good Neighbor
Echinacea, Iron
Bergen Brunswig Drug Company
www.mygnp.com
714-385-4000

Greatest Vitamin in the World
Multivitamins
The Greatest Vitamin in the World
www.thegreatestvitamininthe world.com
800-605-VITA

More Brand Information

Health Asure
Vitamin C
Health Asure
www.rainbowlight.com
800-635-1233

Health From the Sun
Cholestrol Lowering, Seed Oils
Health From the Sun
www.healthfromthesun.com
800-447-2229

Health Yourself
Melatonin
HVL, Inc.
www.douglaslabs.com
800-245-4440

Healthy Moments
B Vitamins, Multivitamins
Momentus Solutions, LLC

Healthy Origins
CoQ10
Healthy Origins
www.healthyorigins.com
888-228-6650

Healthy Woman
Menopause
McNeil Consumer Healthcare
www.healthywoman.net/
soy_menopause/
800-962-5357

Herbal Select
Cancer Prevention
Herbal Select
www.herbalselect.com
519-837-2141

Herbalife
*Garlic, Nutrition Powder,
Prostate*
Herbalife
www.herbalife.com
866-866-4744

Hero Nutritionals
Multivitamins
Hero Nutritional Products
www.heronutritionals.com
800-500-4376

Hi-Ener-G
Ginseng
Windmill Health Products
www.windmillvitamins.com
800-822-4320

Himalaya
Garlic
Himalaya USA
www.himalayausa.com
800-869-4640

Hsu's Root to Health
Ginseng
Hsu's Ginseng Enterprises, Inc.
www.hsuginseng.com
800-826-1577

HydraJoint
Joint Care
Renutra Natural Health Products
www.hydrajoint.com
877-834-2377

Imagilin Technology
Probiotics (Pets)
Imagilin Technology, LLC
www.imagilin.com
301-983-5888

Imperial Elixir
Ginseng
GINCO International
www.ginsengcompany.com
800-284-2598

Innovative Natural Products
Melatonin
Innovative Natural Products

Inno-Vite
CoQ10
Inno-Vite
www.inno-vite.com

Iosat
Nuclear Radiation
Anbex, Inc.
www.anbex.com
866-463-6754

Iovate Health Sciences
Muscular Enhancement
Iovate Health Sciences USA Inc.

Iron-Tek
Muscular Enhancement
Iron-Tek
www.iron-tek.com

Irwin Naturals
Memory
Irwin Naturals
www.irwinnaturals.com
800-297-3273

ISS Research
Muscular Enhancement,
Nutrition Powders
ISS Research
www.issresearch.com
888-231-2684

Jamieson
Garlic, Magnesium, Valerian
Jamieson Laboratories
www.jamiesonlabs.com
800-265-5088

Jarrow Formulas
Cancer Prevention, Menopause,
Probiotics, SAMe, Seed Oils,
Jarrow Formulas, Inc.
www.jarrow.com
800-726-0886

Joint Max
Joint Care
Pet Health Solutions
www.jointmax.com
887-564-6862

Kaire
Bone Health, Cholesterol
Lowering
Kaire.com Inc.
www.kaire.com
877-603-1710

Kal
Cancer Prevention, Magnesium,
Menopause, Probiotics, SAMe
Nutraceutical Corp.
www.nutraceutical.com
800-579-4665

Karuna
Joint Care, Memory
Karuna Corporation
www.karunahealth.com
800-711-6740

Kashi
Nutrition Bar
Kashi Company
www.kashi.com
858-274-8870

Keto Bars
Nutrition Bar
Keto Foods and Snacks, Inc.
www.wellfx.com/Shop/Static/
keto-bar.htm
888-624-6240

KI4U
Nuclear Radiation
KI4U Inc.
www.KI4U.com
830-672-8734

More Brand Information

Kinetana
   Ginseng
   Biogenesis Nutraceuticals Inc.
   www.bio-genesis.com
   866-272-0500

Kira
   St. John's Wort
   ABKIT Inc.
   www.lichtwer.com
   800-226-6227

Kirkland
   Joint Care, Multivitamin,
   Omega-3
   Costco Wholesale Corporation
   www.costco.com
   800-774-2678

Kroger
   Valerian
   The Kroger Co.
   www.kroger.com
   866-221-4141

Kwai
   Garlic
   ABKIT, Inc
   www.abkit.com
   800-226-6227

Kyolic
   Garlic, Menopause, Probiotics
   Wakunaga of America
   www.kyolic.com
   800-421-2998

Lane Labs
   Bone Health
   Lane Labs-US, Inc.
   www.lanelabs.com
   800-526-3005

Lean System7
   Weight Loss
   Isatori LLC

www.isatoritech.com
866-688-7679

Libido Max
   Sexual Enhancement
   Applied Nutrition
   www.appliednutrition.com

Life Enhancement
   Memory
   Life Enhancement Products, Inc.
   www.life-enhancement.com
   800-543-3873

Life Extension
   Cancer Prevention, Cholesterol
   Lowering, Chromium,
   Magnesium, Menopause, SAMe
   Life Extension Foundation
   www.lef.org
   800-678-8989

life-flo
   Menopause
   life-flo
   www.life-flo.com
   888-999-7440

LifeTime
   Vitamin C
   Lifetime
   www.lifetimevitamins.com
   800-333-6168

LifeWise Naturals
   Alpha-Lipoic Acid, Bone Health,
   Cholesterol Lowering, Garlic
   LifeWise Naturals, Inc.
   www.lifewise.com
   800-643-9558

Li'l Critters
   Bone Health
   Northwest Natural Products Inc.
   www.gummybearvitamins.com
   800-661-2736

Liquid Calcium
Magnesium
Integrative Therapeutics Inc.
www.integrativeinc.com
800-931-1709

Longs
CoQ10, Magnesium
Longs Drug Stores
www.longs.com
800-421-1168

Lorna Vanderhaeghe SleepSense
Melatonin
Preferred Nutrition
www.healthmart2000.com
888-249-0990

Mason Vitamins
B Vitamins, Garlic, Vitamin E
Mason Vitamins, Inc.
www.masonvitamins.com
800-327-6005

Maxi Health
*Joint Care, Memory, Vitamin C,
Vitamin E*
MaxiHealth Research Inc.
www.maxihealth.com
800-895-9555

The Medicine Shoppe
Potassium
Medicine Shoppe International
www.medicineshoppe.com

Medical Corps
Nuclear Radiation
Medical Corps
www.medicalcorps.com
610-633-2276

MegaFood
Chromium
MegaFood
www.megafood.com

Melatonin Sleep
Melatonin
Northwest Natural Products Inc.
800-661-2736

Member's Mark
Multivitamins, Vitamin C
SWC (Sam's Club)
www.samsclub.com
888-746-7726

Metabolic
Cancer Prevention
Metabolic Maintenance Products
www.metabolicmaintenance.
com
800-772-7873

Metagenics
CLA, Omega-3, Weight Loss
Metagenics, Inc.
www.metagenics.com
800-692-9400

MET-Rx
Nutrition Bar, Nutrition Powder
MET-Rx USA
www.metrx.com
800-556-3879

MHP
Muscular Enhancement
MHP INC.
www.maxperformance.com

More Brand Information

MRM
Alpha-Lipoic Acid, Memory,
Muscular Enhancement,
St. John's Wort
Metabolic Response Modifiers
www.mrm-usa.com
800-948-6296

Muscle Marketing USA
Muscular Enhancement
Muscle Marketing USA
www.mmusa.com
888-332-2501

Muscletech
Muscular Enhancement,
Nutrition Bar, Nutrition Powder
MuscleTech Research and
Development Inc.
www.muscletech.com
888-334-4448

Natrol
CLA, DHEA, Garlic, Iron,
Omega-3, SAMe, Sexual
Enhancers, Weight Loss
Natrol, Inc.
www.natrol.com
800-326-1520

Naturade
Nutrition Powder
Naturade Inc.
www.naturade.com

Natural Balance
Melatonin
Natural Balance, Inc.
www.naturalbalance.com
800-833-8737

Natural Factors
Alpha-Lipoic Acid, B Vitamins,
Magnesium, Potassium,
Probiotics, Zinc
Natural Factors Nutritional
Products Ltd.
www.naturalfactors.com
800-322-8704

Natural Max
CLA, Weight Loss
Nutraceutical Corp.
www.nutraceutical.com
800-669-8877

Nature Made
B Vitamins, Bone Health,
Cancer Prevention, Cholesterol
Lowering, CoQ10, Joint Care,
Melatonin, Menopause,
Magnesium, SAMe, Sight
Enhancement, Vitamin C,
Vitamin E, Zinc
Nature Made Nutritional
Products/Pharmavite
www.NatureMade.com
800-276-2878

Nature's Actives
Menopause
Nutrition Warehouse
www.nutritionwarehouse.com
800-228-4533

Nature's Answer
Cancer Prevention, Valerian,
Vitamin C
Nature's Answer
www.naturesanswer.com
800-439-2324

Nature's Apothecary
Milk Thistle, Valerian
Nature's Apothecary
www.nowfoods.com
886-669-3663

Nature's Bounty
Alpha-Lipoic Acid, B Vitamins,
Bone Health, Cancer Prevention,
CoQ10, DHEA, Magnesium,
Melatonin, Memory, Menopause,
Milk Thistle, Multivitamins,
Omega-3, Prostate, Seed Oils,
Sexual Enhancement, Sight
Enhancement, St. John's Wort,
Vitamin C, Weight Loss
Nature's Bounty, Inc.
www.naturesbounty.com
800-433-2990

Nature's Formulary
Cholesterol Lowering
Nature's Formulary, LLC
www.naturesformulary.com
800-923-9338

Nature's Harmony
Sexual Enhancement
Purity Life Health Products Ltd.
www.naturesharmony.us
888-458-6003

Nature's Life
Alpha-Lipoic Acid, B-Vitamins
Nature's Life
www.natlife.com
800-247-6997

Nature's Plus
Iron, Joint Care, Memory,
Multivitamins, Nutrition Powder
Natural Organics, Inc.
www.naturesplus.com
631-293-0030

Nature's Resource
Echinacea, Garlic, Ginseng,
Menopause, Milk Thistle, St.
John's Wort, Valerian
Nature's Resource Products/
Pharmavite
www.naturesresource.com
800-423-2405

Nature's Secret
Probiotics
Nature's Secret
www.naturessecret.com
800-297-3273

Nature's Sunshine
CLA, Probiotics
Nature's Sunshine Products, Inc.
www.naturessunshine.com
800-223-8225

Nature's Valley
Milk Thistle, Valerian
Albertson's
www.albertsons.com

Nature's Way
Echinacea, Milk Thistle,
Probiotics, Seed Oils, Valerian
Nature's Way Products, Inc.
www.naturesway.com
800-926-8883

Nestle (Carnation)
Nutrition Powders & Drinks
Nestle USA Inc.
www.carnationinstantbreakfast
.com

New Chapter
Chromium, Garlic, Saw Palmetto,
St. John's Wort
New Chapter, Inc.
www.new-chapter.com
800-543-7279

More Brand Information

NEWtritional Defense
Iron
Marlyn-Nutraceuticals, Inc.
www.naturallyvitamins.com
800-899-4499

Nikken
Garlic
Nikken, Inc.
www.nikken.com

Nitro FX
Banned Substances
Enliven International, Inc.
www.enliveninternational.com
800-548-5746

NOW
Magnesium, Melatonin,
Multivitamins, Nutrition Powder,
Prostate, Saw Palmetto, Vitamin C
NOW Foods
www.nowfoods.com
630-545-9098

Nordic Naturals
Omega-3
Nordic Natural, Inc.
www.nordicnaturals.com/
888-662-2544

NSI
Joint Care, Milk Thistle
Nutraceutical Sciences Institute
www.vitacots.com
800-381-0759

Nutralife
SAMe
Nutralife Health Products, Inc.
www.nutralife.com
877-688-7254

Nutravite
Alpha-Lipoic Acid, Memory,
Probiotics
Nutravite Pharmaceuticals
www.nutravite.com
800-416-0911

Nutri Magic
Garlic
Nutri Magic Systems
International Inc.
www.nutrimagic.com
800-401-7096

NutriCology
Potassium, Prostate
NutriCology, Inc.
www.nutricology.com
800-545-9960

Nutrilite
Bone Health, CLA, Chromium,
Echinacea, Garlic, Memory,
Menopause, Milk Thistle,
Multivitamins, Nutrition Bar,
Nutrition Powder, Omega-3,
Probiotic, Prostate, Seed Oils,
Sight Enhancement, Valerian,
Vitamin E
Access Business Group
International
www.nutrilite.com/www.quixtar
.com
800-253-6500

Nutrition Now
Bone Health, Probiotics
Nutrition Now
www.nutritionnow.com
800-929-0418

Nutri-Vet Nutritionals
Joint Care, Seed Oils
Nutri-Vet, LLC
www.nutri-vet.com
877-729-8668

Oakmont Labs
Seed Oils
Oakmont Labs

OCU-MAX
Sight Enhancement
TheraCeuticals Internationals
www.gvi.com
800-535-9816

Olay
Omega-3
Pharmavite LLC
www.olayvitamins.com
800-710-6529

Olympian Labs
Cholesterol Lowering, Memory,
Menopause, SAMe
Olympian Laboratories, Inc.
www.olympianlabs.com
800-473-5883

Omega Brite
Omega-3
Omega Natural Health
www.omegabrite.com
800-383-2030

One-A-Day
Bone Health, Multivitamins
Bayer Corporation
www.oneaday.com
800-331-4536

151 Energy
Nutrition Bar
Applied Nutrition
www.appliednutritioncorp.com/
800-605-0410

One Source
Multivitamins
Perrigo Company
269-673-7962

Only Natural
DHEA
Only Natural, Inc.

Oona
Menopause
Oona
www.oonausa.com
888-596-5154

Optimum Nutrition
Multivitamin, Nutrition Powder
Optimum Nutrition
www.optimumnutrition.com
630-236-0097

Organika
Bone Health, Milk Thistle
Organika Health Products Inc.
www.organika.com
604-277-3302

Origin
Milk Thistle, Omega-3, Vitamin E
Target Corporation
www.target.com
800-440-0680

Paradise Herbs
Ginseng
Paradise Herbs, Inc.
www.paradiseherbs.com
800-691-2573

PatentLean
Weight Loss
PatentHealth LLC
www.patenthealth.com
800-777-8988

Pet-Tabs
Multivitamins
Virback AH, Inc.
www.pfizerah.com
800-366-5288

More Brand Information

Pharmanex
*Alpha-Lipoic Acid, B Vitamins,
Cancer Prevention, Ginseng,
Joint Care, Melatonin,
Multivitamins, Probiotics,
Valerian, Vitamin C, Vitamin E*
Pharmanex
www.pharmanex.com
800-487-1000

Pharm Assure
Memory, Vitamin E
PharmAssure/Rite Aid
Corporation
www.riteaid.com
800-748-3243

Physiologics
DHEA, Prostate
Physiologics
www.physiologics.com

PhytoPharmica
Omega-3, Weight Loss
PhytoPharmica
www.PhytoPharmica.com
800-553-2370

Pinnacle
*Sexual Enhancement, Weight
Loss*
Bodyonics
www.pinnaclebody.com
800-899-2749

Pioneer
B Vitamins, Vitamin C
Pioneer Nutritional Formulas,
Inc.
www.pioneernutritional.com
800-458-8483

Planetary Formulas
Echinacea, Sexual Enhancement
Planetary Formulas
www.planetaryformulas.com
800-606-6226

PowerBar
Nutrition Bar
PowerBar, Inc.
www.powerbar.com
800-587-6937

Prairie Naturals
Vitamin C
Prairie Naturals Health Products
Inc.

Precision Engineered
*Muscular Enhancement,
Nutrition Powder*
U.S. Nutrition
www.vitaminworld.com
800-228-4533

The Premier
Seed Oil
CAG Functional Foods
www.culturelle.com
888-828-4242

Pria
Nutrition Bar
Powerbar, Inc.
www.powerbar.com
800-587-6937

PL
Sexual Enhancement
Progressive Laboratories, Inc.

Pro Health
CoQ10, Memory
Pro Health Inc.
www.prohealth.com
800-366-6056

Promax
Nutrition Bar
Promax Nutrition, Inc.
www.promaxnutrition.net
888-728-8962

Promensil
Menopause
Novogen
www.promensil.com
877-417-7663

Prostate 51X
Prostate
New Chapter, Inc.
www.new-chapter.com
800-543-7279

ProstraPro
Prostate
PhytoPharmica
www.phytopharmica.com
800-376-7889

Pure Encapsulations
Alpha-Lipoic Acid, Garlic, Potassium, St. John's Wort
Pure Encapsulations, Inc.
www.purecaps.com
800-753-2277

Pure Protein
Nutrition Bar
Worldwide Sports Nutrition
www.sportnutrition.com
800-205-9161

Puritan's Pride
Alpha-Lipoic Acid, B Vitamins, Bone Health, Cancer Prevention, Cholesterol Lowering, CoQ10, DHEA, Echinacea, Ginseng, Iron, Joint Care, Magnesium, Melatonin, Memory, Menopause, Milk Thistle, Multivitamins, Muscular Enhancement, Nutrition Powder, Omega-3, Prostate, Seed Oils, Sexual Enhancement, Sight Enhancement, St. John's Wort, Valerian, Vitamin C, Vitamin E, Weight Loss, Zinc

Puritan's Pride, Inc.
www.puritan.com
800-645-1030

Quest
Melatonin
Quest Vitamins
www.questvitamins.com
888-264-0611

Quigley's
Zinc
Quigley Corporation
www.quigleyco.com
800-505-2653

Rad Block
Nuclear Radiation
USDPI

Rainbow Light
Menopause, Weight Loss
Rainbow Light Nutritional Systems
www.rainbowlight.com
800-635-1233

Rexall
B Vitamins, Magnesium, Milk Thistle, Omega-3, Sight Enhancement
Rexall, Inc.
www.rexallsundown.com
888-848-2435

Rite Aid
B Vitamins, CoQ10, Iron, Potassium, Probiotics
Rite Aid Corporation
www.riteaid.com
800-748-3243

Royal King
Ginseng
Herba Natural Products Inc.
www.herbanatural.com
718-832-6929

More Brand Information

Ruger Chemical
Nuclear Radiation
Ruger Chemical Co., Inc.
www.rugerchemical.com
800-274-7843

Rx Vitamins
Cholesterol Lowering
Rx Vitamins, Inc,
www.rxvitamins.com
800-792-2222

Safeway
Iron, Magnesium
Safeway
www.safeway.com
877-723-3929

Sav-on
Omega-3
Albertsons Inc.
www.sav-ondrugs.com
888-746-7252

Schiff
Bone Health, Cancer Prevention, Joint Care, Magnesium, Menopause, Vitamin E
Schiff Products
www.schiffvitamins.com
800-526-6251

SciFit
Muscular Enhancement
SciFit

Shaklee
CoQ10, Seed Oils, Vitamin C, Vitamin E, Valerian
Shaklee
www.shaklee.com
800-742-5533

SISU
B Vitamins, Seed Oils
SISU, Inc.
www.sisuhealth.com
800-663-4163

Skin Formula 3V
Omega-3
DVM Pharmaceuticals
www.dvmpharmaceuticals.com

Slim-Fast
Nutrition Powder
Slim-Fast Foods Company
www.slim-fast.com

Slo Niacin
B Vitamins
Upsher-Smith Laboratories, Inc.
www.upsher-smith.com
800-654-2299

Slow Fe
Iron
Novartis Consumer Health, Inc.
www.novartis.com
800-452-0051

Slow-Mag
Magnesium
Purdue Products L.P.
www.slo-mag.com
888-726-7535

Smart Basics
DHEA, Milk Thistle
Vitacost.com
www.vitacost.com
800-381-0759

Snickers
Nutrition Bar
Masterfoods USA
www.snickers.com

Solaray
*DHEA, Memory, Menopause,
St. John's Wort, Weight Loss*
Nutraceutical Corp.
www.nutraceutical.com
800-579-4665

Solgar
*Alpha-Lipoic Acid, Garlic,
Nutrition Powder, Vitamin E*
Solgar Vitamin and Herb
www.solgar.com
877-765-4274

Source Naturals
*Alpha-Lipoic Acid, Magnesium,
Omega-3, Prostate, Sexual
Enhancement, St. John's Wort*
Source Naturals, Inc.
www.sourcenaturals.com
800-815-2333

Soy Care
Menopause
Inverness Medical, Inc.
www.invernessmedical.com
800-899-7353

Spectrum Essential
ALA
Spectrum Essential
http://www.spectrumorganics.
com

Spring Valley
*CoQ10, Garlic, Ginseng,
Menopause, Milk Thistle,
Omega-3, Prostate, Sight
Enhancing, St. John's Wort,
Vitamin C, Vitamin E*
Wal-Mart
www.walmart.com

St. Ives
Vitamin E
St. Ives Laboratories
www.stives.com

Standard Process Inc.
Bone Health
Standard Process Inc.
www.standardprocess.com
800-848-5061

Sundown
*B Vitamins, Bone Health,
CoQ10, Echinacea, Ginseng,
Iron, Magnesium, Melatonin,
Menopause, Milk Thistle,
Omega-3, Potassium, Prostate,
Seed Oils, Sight Enhancement,
St. John's Wort, Vitamin C,
Vitamin E, Weight Loss*
Rexall Sundown, Inc.
www.sundownnutrition.com
888-848-2435

Sunkist
Zinc
WN Pharmaceuticals, Inc.
www.sunkistvitamins.com
800-430-7898

Sunsource
Garlic, Melatonin
Chattem, Inc.
www.sunsource.com

Swanson
*Ginseng, Joint Care, Menopause,
Multivitamin, Omega-3*
Swanson Health Products
www.swansonvitamins.com
800-603-3198

Swiss Natural Sources
*B Vitamin, Potassium, Valerian,
Vitamin C*
Swiss Herbal Remedies
www.swissherbal.ca
800-268-9879

More Brand Information

Symtec
Joint Care
Symtec Laboratories
www.symteclab.com
800-232-4005

Tahitian Noni Juice
Banned Substances
Tahitian Noni International
www.TahitianNoni.com
801-234-1000

TerraVita
Prostate, Saw Palmetto
TerraVita

Thermosculpt
Chromium, Weight Loss
4 Your Health
www.4YH.com
888-611-5678

Think Thin
Nutrition Bar
Prime Health Dietary
Supplements, Inc.
www.thinkproducts.com
866-988-4465

Thompson
Alpha-Lipoic Acid, Potassium,
Vitamin C, Valerian
Nutraceutical Corp.
www.nutraceutical.com
800-579-4665

Thorne Research
B Vitamins, Zinc
Thorne Research, Inc. (Julian
Whittaker)
www.thorne.com
208-263-1337

Tishcon
CoQ10, Probiotics
Tishcon Corp.
www.tishcon.com
516-333-3050

Trace Minerals Research
Zinc
Trace Minerals Research
www.traceminerals.com
800-624-7145

Trader Darwin's
Melatonin, Potassium
Trader Joe's
www.traderjoes.com
626-599-3817

TriMedica
DHEA, Joint Care, Melatonin
TriMedica, Inc.
www.trimedica.com
800-800-8849

Trimspa
Chromium
Trimspa
www.trimspa.com

Triomega
Omega-3
Inverness Medical, Inc.
www.invernessmedical.com

Tropical Oasis
Valerian
Tropical Oasis
www.tropicaloasis.com
800-815-9354

TruNature
Garlic, Ginseng, Memory,
Menopause, Prostate
Costoco Wholesale Corporation
www.costco.com
800-774-2678

21st Century
ALA, St. John's Wort, Valerian
21st Century HealthCare, Inc./
Pet Products
www.21stcenturyvitamins.com

TwinLab
B Vitamins, Bone Health, Joint Care, Melatonin, Multivitamins, Muscular Enhancement, Sexual Enhancement, Weight Loss
Twin Laboratories/IdeaSphere
www.twinlab.com
800-645-5626

Udo's Choice
ALA
Flora, Inc
www.udoerasmus.com

Ultimate Nutrition
CLA, Sexual Enhancement
Ultimate Nutrition, Inc.
www.ultimatenutrition.com
860-409-7100

Unicity
Melatonin
Unicity
www.unicityglobal.com
800-864-2489

Universal Nutrition
Creatine, Muscular Enhancement
Universal Nutrition
www.universalnutrition.com
800-872-0101

USANA
Banned Substances
USANA
www.usana.com
888-950-9595

Viactiv
Bone Health
McNeil Nutritionals
www.viactiv.com
877-842-2843

Vital Nutrients
Nutrition Powder
Vital Nutrients
www.vital-nutrients.com
877-747-9139

Vitaline
SAMe
Integrative Therapeutics, Inc.
www.ritecare.com
866-877-PILL

Vitamin Depot
SAMe
Vitamin Depot
www.vitamindepotonline.com
312-235-2376

Vitamin Power
Menopause, Sight Enhancement
Vitamin Power, Inc.
www.vitaminpower.com

The Vitamin Shoppe
Alpha-Lipoic Acid, Multivitamins, Omega-3, Prostate, Seed Oils, Weight Loss
The Vitamin Shoppe
www.vitaminshoppe.com
888-880-3055

More Brand Information

Vitamin World
*Alpha-Lipoic Acid, B Vitamins,
Bone Health, Cancer Prevention,
CLA, Cholesterol Lowering,
CoQ10, DHEA, Echinacea,
Ginseng, Iron, Joint Care,
Magnesium, Melatonin,
Memory, Menopause, Milk
Thistle, Multivitamins, Muscular
Enhancement, Nutrition Powder,
Omega-3, Potassium, Prostate,
Seed Oils, Sexual Enhancement,
Sight Enhancing, St. John's Wort,
Valerian, Vitamin C, Vitamin E,
Weight Loss, Zinc*
Vitamin World, Inc.
www.vitaminworld.com
631-244-2125

Vitanica
CoQ10, Menopause
Vitanica
www.vitanica.com
800-572-4712

VitaSmart
*CoQ10, Potassium, Prostate,
Vitamin C*
Kmart
www.kmart.com
866-562-7848

Vita-Treat
Probiotics (Pets)
Vita-Treat
www.vitatreat.com

Vitol Products
Muscle Enhancement
Vitol Products, Inc.

Walgreens
*Ginseng, Joint Care, Magnesium,
Prostate, Vitamin E*
Walgreens
www.walgreens.com
800-289-2273

Webber Naturals
*Joint Care, Menopause,
Probiotics*
WN pharmaceuticals, Inc.
www.webbernaturals.com
800-430-7898

Weil Nutritional Supplements
Joint Care, Multivitamins
Weil Lifestyle, LLC
www.drweil.com

Wellness International
DHEA
Wellness International Network,
Ltd.
www.web.winltd.com
972-312-1100

Whole Foods
*Cancer Prevention, Echinacea,
Magnesium, Menopause,
Omega-3*
Whole Foods Market
www.wholefoodsmarket.com
512-477-4455

Wild Oats
Memory, Menopause
Wild Oats Markets, Inc.
www.wildoats.com
800-494-9453

Windmill
Ginseng, Vitamin E
Windmill Vitamin Co, Inc.
www.windmillvitamins.com
800-822-4320

WinFuel
Multivitamins
WinFuel, Inc.
www.winfuel.com
800-9-WINFUEL

Winn-Dixie
Potassium
Winn-Dixie
www.winndixie.com
866-946-6349

Woman's Wellbeing
Menopause
Consumer Choice Systems, Inc.

Worldwide Sports Nutrition
Nutrition Powders
Worldwide, Inc.
www.sportsnutrition.com
800-205-9161

WynnPharm
Joint Supplement
Rotta Pharmaceuticals, Inc.
www.wynnpharm.com
800-214-9600

XanGo
Banned Substances
XanGo, LLC
www.xango.com
888-939-2646

Xenadrine
Weight Loss
Cytodyne
www.xenadrine.com
888-Cytodyne

XS
Nutrition Bar
Access Business Group
www.quixtarenergybar.com/
800-253-6500

Zand
Milk Thistle, Zinc
Zand Herbal Formulas
www.zand.com
800-232-4005

Zantrex
Weight Loss
Zoller Labs
www.zollerlabs.com
800-392-3689

Zone Perfect
Omega-3, Nutrition Powder
Zone Perfect Nutrition Company
www.zoneperfect.com
800-390-6690

Index

Index

Index

Index

Index

Product Index

Product Index

Product Index

Product Index

Product Index

Product Index

Product Index

Product Index